Lessons from a
Disabled Caregiver

Lessons from a Disabled Caregiver

*Thriving Together and Maintaining
Independence with Physical
Disability and Dementia*

WILLIAM G. REED

Foreword by MARWAN NOEL SABBAGH, M.D.

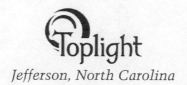

Toplight

Jefferson, North Carolina

LIBRARY OF CONGRESS CATALOGUING-IN-PUBLICATION DATA

Names: Reed, William G., 1941– author.
Title: Lessons from a disabled caregiver : thriving together
and maintaining independence with physical disability and dementia /
William G. Reed ; foreword by Marwan Noel Sabbagh, M.D.
Description: Jefferson, North Carolina : Toplight, 2021 |
Includes bibliographical references and index.
Identifiers: LCCN 2021024156 | ISBN 9781476687391 (paperback : acid free paper) ∞
ISBN 9781476645216 (ebook)
Subjects: LCSH: Reed, William G., 1941- | People with disabilities—
United States—Biography | Male caregivers—United States—Biography. |
Alzheimer's disease—Patients—Care—United States. | Alzheimer's disease—
Patients—Family relationships—United States. | Caregivers—United States—
Conduct of life. | BISAC: MEDICAL / Caregiving
Classification: LCC HV1553 .R435 2021 | DDC 362.4092—dc23
LC record available at https://lccn.loc.gov/2021024156

BRITISH LIBRARY CATALOGUING DATA ARE AVAILABLE

ISBN (print) 978-1-4766-8739-1
ISBN (ebook) 978-1-4766-4521-6

On the cover: The author works on publishing this book
with loving support from his wife photograph by Sade' Bundy

Printed in the United States of America

Toplight is an imprint of McFarland & Company, Inc., Publishers

*Box 611, Jefferson, North Carolina 28640
www.toplightbooks.com*

*I dedicate this book to the memory of my mother,
Evelyn Hower Reed, who died from lung cancer too soon,
and my father, Frank Hibbs Reed, who provided a strong moral
example for us as he played the roles of mother and father.
Most of all, I dedicate this book to Joan Derby Reed,
who has been my loving wife for more than 54 years.*

"*Difficulties and adversities viciously force all their might on us ... they are necessary elements of individual growth and reveal our true potential. We have got to endure and overcome them, and move forward. Never lose hope. Storms make people stronger and never last forever.*"

—Roy T. Bennett, *The Light in the Heart*

Table of Contents

Foreword
by Marwan Noel Sabbagh, M.D.

I am a medical doctor, a neurologist, who has dedicated his whole career to diagnosing, treating, and managing patients with Alzheimer's disease dementia (AD), other dementias, and memory disorders. In order to maintain objectivity, I try to take a dispassionate approach as a physician. However, even with the external appearance of the stolid clinician, I cannot help but feel moved by patient, life, and caregiver experiences. At the end of the day, we are all just people with our own life experiences, relationships, families, struggles and triumphs.

In this helpful guide, we learn about Bill Reed's very emotional story. The story converges the autobiographical experience of Bill's long term physical disability and his being the caregiver to his wife of more than five decades with practical, real-life recommendations for caring for a loved one suffering from Alzheimer's dementia. He provides extensive references that will be helpful to those dealing with physical disability and those caring for dementia patients.

At the top level, it is a story of "love conquers all" that is the driver for Bill's care of Jodie. Deeper within the story is a case study of resilience. *Merriam Webster* defines resilience as "1: the capability of a strained body to recover its size and shape after deformation caused especially by compressive stress. 2: an ability to recover from or adjust easily to misfortune or change." It is the second definition that applies to caregiving. Wikipedia defines psychological resilience as "the ability to mentally or emotionally cope with a crisis or to return to pre-crisis status quickly." Resilience exists when the person uses "mental processes and behaviors in promoting personal assets and protecting self from the potential negative effects of stressors."

The story of Bill and Jodie Reed is a case study of physical and psychological resilience. Although love is enduring, the day-to-day challenges of physical disability and caregiver stress are difficult to endure day in and day out. Caregiving by its nature is exhausting as the caregiver steps in to manage a loved one who is suffering from AD. This includes managing finances, assisting with Activities of Daily Living (ADLs), offsetting behavioral issues, and the list goes on and on. A caregiver assumes living two lives and not one. It is tiring even when it is going well and physical disability of the caregiver is not present. What is important here is that the author is taking a practical approach in the book with his recommendations on how to administer caregiving in the face of physical disability. The story itself is both inspiring and informative and practical. Often there is no "how-to" manual on caregiving in dementia. This is a very good version of a "how-to" manual. I found it a worthy read and I hope you do too.

Marwan Noel Sabbagh, M.D., a board-certified neurologist and geriatric neurologist, is considered one of the leading experts in Alzheimer's and dementia. He holds the Camille and Larry Ruvo Endowed Chair for Brain Health and is the director of the Cleveland Clinic Lou Ruvo Center for Brain Health in Las Vegas. He has authored and coauthored more than 320 medical and scientific articles on Alzheimer's research and has been recognized with numerous awards.

Preface

"...for every disability you have, you are blessed with more than enough abilities to overcome your challenges."
—Nick Vujicic, Australian Christian evangelist and motivational speaker

This is an experience-based book designed to help those living with life-altering medical conditions and/or those dealing with challenging caregiving responsibilities. Its purpose is to help people in those situations find solutions to the challenges they face. I am dealing with both.

Untreatable progressive muscle and nerve diseases have transformed me from an athlete into someone dependent on a wheelchair and specialized equipment for all of life's activities. But my primary responsibility is caring for my wife, Jodie, who has Alzheimer's.

I had not considered writing a book until my daughter, Kris, suggested it. Having seen the numerous obstacles I have overcome, she and several other people strongly encouraged me to share what I have learned so that others could benefit from my journey. As I advanced through many stages of progressive disease, I have confronted a multitude of problems. The solutions I found will help those suffering from chronic debilitating medical conditions. Individuals disabled from a car accident or a surgery that went wrong can also gain insight into how to cope with their limitations. This book demonstrates that you can overcome your challenges, maintain your independence, and have a happy, fulfilling life.

My objective is to assist as many people as possible. To accomplish this goal, I have provided numerous references, so those in situations that differ from my own can also find solutions. The purpose of providing this information is to help ensure that you have a better quality of life and can maintain your independence as long as possible. Your experience will not be identical to mine, but you will face similar issues. For situations that differ in some details, the references provided will expand and broaden your knowledge base.

I do not claim to be an expert on any of the subjects I cover in this book and have not tried to be comprehensive on all subject matter. I draw on my personal experience and include pictures to discuss various solutions, safety concerns, and details about problems you may encounter and the decisions you will have to make. I have also provided cost information to help in your decision-making.

I started writing this book in April 2019 and completed it in June 2020. A broken leg in July 2020 and related issues discussed in the Epilogue delayed my search for a publisher for several months. I delivered the manuscript to Toplight, an imprint of McFarland & Co., in February 2021. The timeline in this paragraph is important because my wife's condition and my own continually change. Except in the Epilogue, changes that occurred after June 2020 are generally not included.

In addition to the dates mentioned above, I have provided other dates for key events to give you a sense of our situation at any given time. The timeline indicates how fast things changed. For example, how long was a walker a safe mobility device before an equipment change was needed?

Because of these changes, the situation described in one chapter may not be the case in a subsequent chapter. For example, initially, I can drive, then can't, then can again with a specialized vehicle and controls. To minimize confusion, I use parentheses to note such changes. For example, I wrote Chapter 13, Stand and Transfer Safely, when we lived in our home in California, but before I finished the book, we lived in a retirement community in Arizona where I acquired a hospital bed. I included information about the hospital bed in parentheses.

The flow of the book is based on the sequence of the major challenges we faced. As a result, caregiving is near the end of the book because caregiving became the biggest issue of our lives then. When I started writing this book in April 2019, my caregiving responsibilities were manageable. My primary focus was on the physical challenges I was encountering. So I wrote sections of the book about those aspects first. But then life happened!

Those personal concerns were eclipsed by the precipitous cognitive decline of my wife into Alzheimer's. By July 2019, our lives were rapidly changing in unexpected ways. I sent the following email to my family on July 10, 2019.

> *Things I have observed about Jodie's status have convinced me that being her caregiver has to expand now and supersede everything. That is going to be my primary focus in ways I had not fully understood until now. She is extremely happy currently, but to maintain that means I need to find new and better ways to care for her.*

Before I started writing this book, I created a preliminary Table of Contents to guide me through the process. It included a section on caregiving with a chapter on senior living. I had no clue we would be living in such a facility by that November. By then I could no longer adequately care for Jodie in our home. Nor did I expect to be caregiving from a wheelchair.

But that is the nature of progressive disease, and it was happening to both of us, especially my wife, at an alarming rate. Those with a diagnosis of progressive disease, be it physical or mental, must expect significant changes and attempt to be ready for them. Our experience might help you prepare for the future.

The book starts with your discovery that you have a severe medical condition and your possible reaction to this life-changing news. The rest of the book is about accepting and adapting to your new and changing circumstances while maintaining a productive, independent life. It concludes with chapters about caregiving for Alzheimer's and dementia patients and senior living. The Epilogue describes the tragedies that occurred after the body of the book was written and how we dealt with them.

The appendices include other useful information, including the types of senior living facilities available, long-term care insurance, and end-of-life planning, which is vital for those left behind, especially if you are a caregiver for someone experiencing a mental decline.

I had always lived my life believing that if you understand what might happen and plan for it, you can handle it. Concerning my physically debilitating diseases, that has mostly been true. But it did not prove valid when dealing with my wife's sudden changed circumstances. Even careful planning cannot anticipate all possible situations.

I firmly believe that it takes a positive attitude and continual perseverance to navigate through all the seemingly impossible problems that arise. This was true for dealing with my physical issues and my wife's cognition problems.

You will encounter numerous obstacles to achieving your goals. At times, the difficulty and number of challenges will seem overwhelming. But when approaching these challenges with an optimistic attitude, perseverance, and ingenuity, you will gain the power to overcome them and be able to maintain your independence longer. I am a firm believer in self-reliance and being your own advocate. However, you will need a robust support network and to be willing to seek help when needed to persevere through the minefield of problems to maintain a happy, fulfilling life.

Introduction

"The adventure of life is to learn. The purpose of life is to grow. The nature of life is to change. The challenge of life is to overcome. The essence of life is to care. The opportunity of life is to serve. The secret of life is to dare. The spice of life is to befriend. The beauty of life is to give."

—William Arthur Ward

For a book about one subject, e.g., a biography, the Introduction would be relatively short. Frequently, there is no introduction to such books.

But this book covers a broad range of subject matter, all of which is of interest to people experiencing a physical or mental disability. The same is true for those who are caring for a person with disabilities. To adequately cover these subjects, I have included 35 chapters, an epilogue and four appendices. Such a scope requires a more comprehensive Introduction. I have also provided some reviewer comments on each section to give you a sense of its importance and the reviewers' reactions to it.

The following is an overview of the seven sections of the book.

Section One: Life Forever Changed

This section describes the reactions you may have when you realize that you have a serious, progressive medical condition or a sudden loss of capability that will significantly change your life. I provide suggestions for coping with these reactions. Since you may not initially have a complete diagnosis of your condition, I relate the steps I went through to reach my diagnosis.

Reviewer comments: *"This chapter will be valuable to anyone who reads it. I particularly liked the attitudes and life philosophy expressed in: the uselessness of distressing about past decisions which cannot be changed; do now when you can and don't wait as it might be too late later; your examples of grief tug at the heartstrings and draws the reader in in empathy."*

"[E]veryone gets to experience grief somewhere along life's journey … this chapter gives the reader a vicarious experience that will help prepare them for their own."

Section Two: Acceptance and Adaptation

After the initial shock and possible depression associated with learning that your life has changed materially, you must accept the new reality and adapt. Family, social and religious life can provide essential support in this process. Maintaining, even strengthening, your muscles can delay the emergence of new challenges. Finding capable, reliable people to help get essential tasks done will make your life simpler and happier. I explain how these actions helped me.

Reviewer comments: *"The recounting of personal experiences throughout the life cycle allows the reader to reflect on their own circumstances and experiences."*

"You cite the basic truth that family and stable relationships are core and most centrally important to a happy mortal life."

"You provide useful advice here. I think the most valuable part is telling your reader that things will change. They won't be able to do what they can do now. Accept it and prepare for it."

Section Three: Safe Personal Mobility Solutions

Your mobility will be a significant challenge, and the acceptable solutions change over time if you have a progressive disease. I describe the alternative equipment available at each stage, the pros and cons of these choices, and the rationale for my choices.

It can be difficult to get insurance coverage for the necessary equipment. This section includes a step-by-step procedure I developed after experiencing difficulties in getting insurance coverage for medical equipment. Following this procedure will help ensure you get coverage for the specific equipment you want. I have also included a table of codes Medicare will accept.

I discuss the potential need for and use of canes, orthotics, a rolling walker, a motorized scooter, and a motorized wheelchair. I also describe how to deal with house level changes.

Reviewer comments: *"These chapters are specific, personal, and likely to be helpful to a broad range of readers."*

"The amount of both effort and research you have put forth on this important writing are amazing.... It will be great to get all this valuable information in the hands of those who need it."

Section Four: Independent Life

You will want to avoid depending on others for the daily activities of life so that you can maintain an independent life as long as possible. Standing up from beds, chairs, and your mobility device, e.g., wheelchair, and transferring to other equipment occurs frequently each day and can be dangerous and risky. The same is true for showering and toiletry. With progressive disease, these challenges increase over time. This section examines the equipment available and the techniques that will allow you to perform these functions independently. In each of these cases, I make specific recommendations and provide descriptive pictures.

When you need a mobility device to shower, you likely will have to modify your bathroom so that you can shower independently. Because of the showering challenge that I faced in my home, I have included pictures of a mock-up of the shower room that I used to verify that my plan would work. Again, equipment recommendations are provided and photographs are included.

Other subjects like preparing for emergencies and acquiring food and supplies when you can't drive are discussed in this section.

> Reviewer comments: *"Your A-to-Z approach, particularly admitting that some decisions could have been different had you thought further ahead, should really get your readers to expand their analysis to include what could and probably will happen with time."*
>
> *"Your thoughts and detailed analyses that are displayed in all your chapters make it easy for readers experiencing various debilitating illnesses to pick and choose what will work best for them."*

Section Five: Vehicle Mobility

Depending on the level of your disability, you may be able to drive an unmodified vehicle for some time but need to transport a motorized mobility device. This section describes how I modified my Sport Utility Vehicle (SUV) to allow me to drive while carrying a motorized scooter. After I could no longer drive, the modified SUV was still essential when someone drove for me. Public transportation options are also included in this section.

> Reviewer comment: *"Very helpful information [on] something that is very important to know about. I am learning much!"*

Section Six: Learning to Drive with Handicaps

When it is no longer possible to drive a standard vehicle, it is still possible for most people to drive using a modified vehicle with controls specifically designed for their condition. There are alternate ways to accomplish this. I explain the approach of being evaluated by a Certified Driver Rehabilitation Specialist to verify that you can drive and to select the optimum controls.

Choosing the right vehicle depends on several factors. Information to help you make the right selection is provided in this section.

Controls installation became an unexpected, disturbing experience for me that affected not only the hand controls but other safety options like blind-spot monitoring. Because five different firms were involved in creating my handicap-equipped van, it became a complicated mystery regarding what happened, who was responsible, and how the issues could be resolved. More than six months after the van delivery, the answers were still not clear. I explain these issues in detail to help you decide who you should hire and whether some of the recommended controls are worth the potential consequences.

Department of Motor Vehicles (DMV) and insurance implications are also discussed in Section Six.

Reviewer comments: *"Fascinating reading, even for one who isn't handicapped."*

"Readers heading down this path should benefit greatly from your experiences and suggestions. Driving is one of the last privileges aging people rely on to preserve their independence."

Section Seven: Caregiving from a Wheelchair

Being a caregiver, particularly for a family member, is a very stressful, time-consuming experience. The challenges that a caregiver must overcome increase dramatically and can be overwhelming when the patient is in mental decline. My challenge was to provide care from a wheelchair for my wife who suffers from Alzheimer's and who is a noncompliant patient, i.e., often unwilling to accept direction and always unwilling to take medication or medical tests.

There are ten chapters in this section. The first four relate my experience as a caregiver in our home and why that became untenable, causing us to move to a senior living facility. I describe what I experienced, the solutions I tried and the effectiveness of them.

Based on the comments I received from my reviewers, these chapters were the most emotionally impactful chapters of the book.

Reviewer comments: *"This is truly amazing writing. I'm blown away. Hits home. So beautiful and heartfelt."*

"I know that this chapter was the hardest for you to write, and honestly, it was hard for me to read. I found it brutally honest, infinitely sad, and courageous."

"Made it thru Chapters 27–29 but just barely. You bared your soul and spared no details.... Very powerful and well composed and the discussion flows smoothly.... Had to be a tough chapter to write but it speaks to the power of love."

"Your chapter on crisis ... reads as if I were living it."

"I cannot find the words to express how it impacted me. I have known a few friends/family with AD and your daughter-in-law's words explains the phenomenon that I felt dealing with the situation."

"I have no words to describe what I felt reading this ... such heartfelt words from your sister-in-law and you! I truly hope I will get to read your book someday...."

"This chapter was absolutely engrossing. I couldn't put it down. Every person that had an experience with this, such as I, even though it was minor and very short term compared to your situation, will feel the same way when they read it."

The middle two chapters explain how we decided to move to a senior care facility and the challenges that had to be overcome to achieve the move quickly.

The final four chapters provide information on senior living's advantages, our social integration, and my wife's adaptation to senior living. The book ends on a positive note as life greatly improved for us due to finding the right medication and senior living advantages.

"Wow! [T]his is a perfect way to end your book! Great work!"

"Excellent work. Love the finish; inspiring and hopeful. Thank you for allowing me to be small part of your endeavor."

Epilogue

The epilogue describes the tragedies that we faced one month after finishing the book. They caused life-altering, permanent changes for us. I describe these changes and how we adjusted to our new circumstances to continue to live happy, joyful lives.

Reviewer comment: *"Great ending!"*

Appendices

Appendix I provides information on the types and costs of senior living facilities that might be available in your area.

Reviewer comments: *"What you have put in the Appendix is great. I am sure it will be an eye-opener for everyone. It will show people what range of service, amenities, and costs are in the industry. It certainly will jog a lot of people to do their homework in preparation for a stay at one of these facilities."*

"What a wealth of information you have included. I doubt that any other reference has as much specific data as you have compiled."

Appendix II describes the advantages and disadvantages of purchasing long-term care insurance.

Appendix III provides a guide for the documents you should create to minimize the stress and difficulty your heirs would otherwise face when you die.

Appendix IV provides ways to ensure that your heirs will have immediate access to the essential documents upon your death.

Reviewer comment: *"You have created a great guideline for everyone to follow."*

In this book I share what I have learned as I declined physically and cared for my wife, who progressed through Alzheimer's ravages. I researched many subjects to learn how to live independently myself and how to care for my wife. This book includes many references that will be useful for those whose challenges are different from mine.

The most important thing I have learned and my overriding message is that a positive attitude and perseverance are essential to your success.

Life Forever Changed

"Any fact facing us is not as important as our attitude toward it, for that determines our success or failure."
—Norman Vincent Peale, in *B & O Magazine* (July 1951)

There are two chapters in this section. The first discusses how I got an early warning that I might have a muscle disease decades before there was any physical evidence to support this concern. It also describes the process I went through to get a final diagnosis when serious symptoms occurred.

The second chapter is about the grief you go through when it becomes clear that you are facing a life-changing diagnosis. It suggests ways to deal with your new reality and associated grief.

1

Recognition and Diagnosis

*"For myself I am an optimist—it does not seem to be much use being
anything else."*

—Winston Churchill, in a speech at the
Lord Mayor's banquet, London, November 9, 1954

A disease could be attacking your nerves or muscles without your knowledge. After taking a blood test in 1992, I was told that I needed to go to the hospital immediately because I might be having a heart attack. It didn't seem logical because I had just completed a vigorous game of basketball. The test showed that I had a high Creatine Kinase (CK) level, 433 percent higher than the high end of normal. There are three types of CK isoenzymes. One is found in the skeletal muscle and heart, another is found in the heart and rises when the heart muscle is damaged, and the third is found mostly in the brain. More tests found that Aldolase, another enzyme in the blood that indicates skeletal muscle damage, was also high.

Usually, these enzymes show up in blunt trauma cases like a car accident but can also result from a muscle disease. As I hadn't had any physical damage, these results suggested there must be damage associated with major skeletal muscles, so I consulted a neurologist. He said that the only way to prove whether I had a muscle disease was to do a biopsy. However, even if the results were negative, that might just mean they didn't biopsy in the right place. In any case, they had no cure even if they could prove I had a muscle disease, so I opted not to have a biopsy. In retrospect, I don't know why they didn't perform Electromyography (EMG) and Nerve Conduction Study (NCS),* tests which I later learned are usually done, but they wouldn't have changed anything.

Nearly twenty years passed before the first physical evidence of disease appeared. I noticed that I had a hard time squeezing a lemon to put lemon juice into my iced tea but didn't recognize the significance. More time passed before I noticed that it was harder to get up from chairs. At an appointment with a rheumatologist for gout, I mentioned that I had trouble getting up from chairs, even though this symptom wasn't associated with my appointment. He asked me to put my arms straight out and stand. I couldn't do it! That shocked me because my legs

---

* A more detailed discussion of these tests is provided later in this chapter.

14

were the strongest part of my body from playing basketball for many years. He sent a note to my General Practitioner (GP) recommending that the cause of this weakness be found.

Soon after this appointment, I suddenly fell face forward. I couldn't understand why but I was hurrying and assumed I caught my foot and stumbled. But it happened again! It seemed that my left leg just gave out.

I had a history of lower back problems and there was a chance that my loss of lower leg strength was caused by spinal stenosis, which is a narrowing of the spaces within your spine. Spinal stenosis is common for people over 50 and is caused by the wear and tear of bones that weaken as you age. Accidents and injuries can also cause stenosis. Stenosis can lead to significant nerve damage affecting your muscles. Various tests confirmed that I did have stenosis, but it wasn't clear that this was the cause and, in retrospect, didn't explain the lemon squeezing issue.

A new neurologist evaluated me with Electromyography (EMG) and Nerve Conduction Study (NCS) tests and concluded that I had Length Dependent Polyneuropathy. Polyneuropathy refers to the form of peripheral neuropathy where many or most of the nerves are affected. According to the NIH National Institute of Neurological Disorders and Stroke,[1]

> More than 20 million people in the United States have been estimated to have some form of peripheral neuropathy, but this figure may be significantly higher—not all people with symptoms of neuropathy are tested for the disease and tests currently don't look for all forms of neuropathy.... About three-fourths of polyneuropathies are "length-dependent," meaning the farthest nerve endings in the feet are where symptoms develop first or are worse. In severe cases, such neuropathies can spread upwards toward the central parts of the body. In non-length dependent polyneuropathies, the symptoms can start more toward the torso, or are patchy.

If you have been diagnosed with nerve disease or muscle disease, you have probably had these tests. They are not pleasant but are necessary to decide whether you have one of these conditions. EMG measures your muscle response (electrical activity) in response to nerve stimulation of the muscle. During the test, needles (electrodes) are inserted into the muscle and electrical activity is picked up and displayed on an oscilloscope. You are measured at rest and different variations of contraction. A person with no nerve or muscle disease would not show any electrical activity at rest.

During an NCS, your nerve is stimulated with electrode patches on your skin, and a "mild" electrical impulse is sent through one of these and the oscilloscope records the result. The different strength impulses don't feel mild! The response speed is determined by the distance between the electrodes and the time it takes for the pulse to travel between them. A neurologist uses the results of these tests to diagnose your condition.

Sometimes it's good to challenge an early diagnosis. My brothers and I played sports in high school and college, so we had worked out most of our lives. Due to my concern about my declining strength, I made notes about what weights I could move with different pieces of equipment and compared them with what my brothers could do. By comparison, I learned that my quads were much weaker than the rest of my body and that the left quad was significantly weaker than the right. I went back to the neurologist and asked whether Length Dependent Polyneuropathy explained the difference in left and right quad strength. The answer was "Maybe not." More tests were done and after consulting with another neurologist, it was concluded that I also had Inclusion Body Myositis (IBM) as well. According to the Muscular Dystrophy Association (MDA),[2]

> Inclusion body myositis (IBM) is one of the most common disabling inflammatory myopathies among patients older than age 50. Based on two small studies conducted in the '80s and '90s, 1 to nearly 8 annual incidences of IBM are expected in every 1 million Americans…. By 15 years, most patients require assistance with basic daily routines, and some become wheelchair-bound or bedridden.

When I looked up IBM symptoms on the Cleveland Clinic website,[3] my reaction was "That's what I have." The first two symptoms listed were "difficulty with gripping, pinching, and buttoning; and weakness of the wrist and finger muscles." This explained why I had such difficulty squeezing lemons and why I was dropping things. The article also said: "Falling and tripping usually are the first noticeable symptoms." Falling wasn't the first symptom I noticed but it was my most serious symptom. They also listed the following symptoms:

1. Atrophy (shrinking or wasting) of the muscles of the forearms.
2. Weakness and visible wasting of the quadriceps muscles. (It was the quads weakness that caused me to challenge the polyneuropathy diagnosis but I knew nothing about IBM at the time.)
3. Weakness of the lower leg muscles, below the knees.
4. Weakness of the esophageal muscles, which can cause dysphagia (difficulty swallowing) in about 30 to 40 percent of patients.*
5. Weakness of other muscle groups as the disease progresses.

My GP asked me to see a physical therapist for swallowing exercises, but I delayed doing that for too long. I now understand why he prescribed this. The MDA article says, "IBM can be an indirect cause of death, mainly due to aspiration pneumonia in patients with difficulty swallowing (dysphagia)."[4] This a good example of when you should not make some of the same decisions I have. Belatedly, I saw a speech therapist who told me I was doing all the right things.

Sharing even little changes in your condition with your doctor might result in an earlier diagnosis and possible treatment. In my case, what I had was untreatable, but knowing what I had would have allowed me to plan ahead sooner. It is best to think long-term if you have a progressively debilitating disease. Short-term solutions may work for a while, but you might have made different decisions if you had been thinking about longer-term issues. In a later chapter, I will discuss the importance of a neurologist diagnosis in getting insurance to cover some or all medical equipment costs.

The next chapter describes the stages of grief you may experience when you learn of your life-altering news and how to deal with them.

---

* I have swallowing issues and I have had to avoid peanut butter for this reason.

2

Dealing with Grief

*"Grief drives men into habits of serious reflection, sharpens the under-
standing and softens the heart."*
—John Adams, in letter to Thomas Jefferson, May 6, 1816

When you first learn that you have a chronic, debilitating condition, you realize that your life has changed materially. This realization is likely to cause you to
experience various stages of grief. There are many resources available to help you
deal with your grief; this chapter will provide some of them.

Elisabeth Kübler-Ross was a psychiatrist and a pioneer in near-death studies. In her groundbreaking book, *On Death and Dying*,[1] she described her theory of the five stages of grief, also known as the "Kübler-Ross Model." The
stages Kübler-Ross identified are denial, anger, bargaining, depression, and
acceptance.

Socialworktoday.com has a much deeper discussion on this subject titled
"Grieving Chronic Illness and Injury—Infinite Losses"[2] by Kate Jackson. I recommend that you read it if you or someone you are caring for is experiencing grief.
Another resource worth reading is *Healing Your Chronic Illness Grief: 100 Practical Ideas for Living Your Best Life*[3] by Jaimie A. Wolfelt and Alan D. Wolfelt, Ph.D.

What is not always recognized or understood is that caregivers experience
these same conditions of grief, in some cases more severely than the patient. If
you are a caregiver or a family member or friend of one, I recommend that you
read "Grief and Loss"[4] by Family Caregiver Alliance and reviewed by Rabbi Jon
Sommer. It details the physical, social, emotional, and spiritual symptoms of caregivers' grief.

Depending on your situation, a physician, psychologist, grief counselor, support group, your religious community, personal research through books and the
Internet, or a combination of these resources are there to provide help.

When you are struggling with grief, friends may suggest valuable resources.
One very meaningful to me is a poem by Charles R. Swindoll[*] titled "Attitude."
My son's father-in-law, Richard, framed it and gave it to me as a Christmas pres-
ent. After reading it to me, he said: "That's you." I strongly agree with his essay's

---

[*] Charles R. Swindoll is an evangelical Christian pastor, author, educator, and radio preacher. He
founded Insight for Living, which airs a radio program on more than 2,000 stations around the world in
15 languages.

message because it is consistent with the philosophy of this book. It is worth reading and can be found on the Internet.*

As we are all individuals dealing with our own specific problems, we react differently to serious issues and need to find alternate ways to deal with them. Like so many who have a health crisis thrust upon them suddenly, I found myself at a loss for readily available information and answers. Hopefully, discussing my own experiences with grief and what family, friends, and acquaintances have told me about their experiences will aid you as you search for help.

Bob Lindsay, one of my fraternity brothers, told me his wife, Pat, suffered a ruptured cerebral aneurysm three years ago. As a result, their lives changed suddenly. As you would expect, they went through various stages of grief. Bob said, "She was one of the 'lucky' ones, but is now suffering the many side effects in a continual decline both mentally and physically. Needless to say it has taken a toll on me. I read books, talked with the medical community, attended support groups, talked with others with similar problems and other caregivers. Some info was helpful, others not so much. I'm still searching and seeking. I wish I had your book three years ago…. We have dealt with inability to do things we always took for granted, downsizing, changing priorities, finding help, a medical community that sometimes is less than helpful, etc., etc."

Larry Haack, another fraternity brother, has a surgery-induced nerve condition and is not healing as hoped. His life changed suddenly, not only because of his physical challenges but also because his wife is dealing with medical challenges. Larry said: "My wife has severe anxiety and depression[.] [A]lthough she is currently controlled with medication, she is developing memory loss." As a result, both Larry and his wife have experienced various stages of grief.

I have seen firsthand the various stages of grief as my wife Jodie has experienced them. When her father died suddenly of a heart attack about 40 years ago while visiting our Maine home, she must have been in shock because she called me at work and stated flatly, "Dad died." I heard no emotion; that was very unlike her. Days later, in a state of denial, she told me that she thought we were driving down to see her dad and family when we were going to her father's funeral.

As so often happens, her mother died shortly after that. Forty years later, due to her progressive dementia, Jodie wanted to call her mother. When I told her that her mother died over 40 years ago, I saw many of the stages of grief. The denial was vehement and the anger palpable because she was sure I was lying. For months, every few days she had to relearn that her mother was gone and grieve again. It has affected me greatly to see her crying and in such pain. She accepted that her mother passed for a time, but it didn't stop her frequent intense sadness when she remembered it. Then in August 2019, I had to tell her that her brother, her last sibling, also died, which caused a similar grief pattern. More recently she again started to think her mother still lives; I usually deflect the conversation to limit her pain without reminding her that her mother is gone.

As for myself, surprisingly, I didn't get overly depressed about the possibility

---

* https://www.inspirationalstories.com/poems/attitude-charles-swindoll-poem/

of muscle disease and its potential impact on my life after getting the initial CK and Aldolase results described in the previous chapter. I believe that was because I was still very healthy and symptoms didn't show up for many years. However, during that period there were many times that I thought I had experienced something that might be the onset of muscle disease. Such worry is non-productive, but there was a positive from my concern. I worked to meet my life goals sooner, which otherwise I might have postponed. For example, I hiked up Mt. Diablo, which is near my home, shortly after I got the news, thinking maybe I wouldn't have a chance later.

Even after I started showing the effects of physical decline, I didn't suffer through many of the stages of grief. I believe that a sudden loss of function caused by a car accident or surgery would have been far more difficult for me. The symptoms of muscle deterioration snuck up on me slowly and I was able to deal with them, so I never was overly distressed. Even when I was told that there was no cure and I would deteriorate over time, I had already assumed and accepted that. I just concentrated on finding out what I needed to do to continue to be as functional as possible. However, my experience might not be typical.

When one gets confirmation of a progressively debilitating disease, it often feels like you are in a race against time to achieve the important items on your bucket list. The best example for me was the trip I took with my son Mike to Africa in 2012. We both watch nature programs, particularly those about African animals. I knew this was probably my last chance to make that trip, and being able to do it with my son was fantastic. He had to help me in many ways, e.g., getting in and out of boats and busses. A year later that trip would have been impossible. That same year Jodie and I went to a family reunion in Niagara Falls. The next year we took a spontaneous trip to Glacier National Park and then a family reunion to San Diego. We were able to make one more international trip to Cornwall, England, but it was clear from the difficulties I had in England that it would be our last.

Jodie and I have taken many great trips but now that travel is impossible, we regret that we didn't do more. The obvious message is that you should not postpone doing those things you always planned to do. Do what you can while you can because circumstances change.

There were other occasions where I was impacted by grief. When I was a freshman in high school, my mother died of lung cancer. I sorely missed her as a part of my life after that. There have been occasions when I recall that awkward moment in the hospital where I thought my reaction to her condition might have hurt or disappointed her. Thirty years later, when my family was watching a movie, there was a scene in which a boy walked into a hospital room to see his very sick mother. I completely lost my composure in front of Jodie and our children. They had never seen me in that state before. When I was writing my memoir, my brother, Jim, sent me a letter my mother sent to us from the hospital. Even at an advanced age, those memories have caused me to have intense emotional reactions.

Another example of grief impacting me was when I received the disturbing news that I had prostate cancer. The tests indicated a high probability that it had already spread, and I immediately experienced grief and depression. Fortunately, they weren't long-lasting. I found the best way to minimize this devastating news' emotional effect was to focus on the best way to treat the disease, identify the best doctor to treat me and focus on my work. After considering surgery, radiation, and hormones, I elected surgery because I wanted that thing out of me! However, there was fear, which led to me choosing a surgeon who was available to operate sooner than one who was better qualified. There were long-lasting and unpleasant after-effects from the surgery that affected my quality of life. Some nerves were cut that left me incontinent and impotent. I struggled with whether the side effects would have been avoided if I had waited for the other surgeon. I tortured myself with negative thoughts for a while. I had to remind myself that the only essential objective was curing my cancer, which had been accomplished. Worrying about past decisions is counterproductive and changes nothing. Later, I had male sling surgery* that almost eliminated urinary incontinence.

One of the challenges of writing a book when both you and your wife have progressive diseases is that your circumstances change and what you wrote a couple of months ago is no longer your status. About three months after the first draft of this chapter was written, by far the most impactful grief I have experienced since my mother died occurred. I had been taking on progressively more care for Jodie over time because she was declining mentally. However, a sudden, rapid change in July 2019 convinced me that being her caregiver had to expand and supersede everything. I was overwhelmed and without answers. She wouldn't go to doctor's appointments, take medicine or submit to routine blood or urine tests, which meant the doctors couldn't provide much help. She rejected anyone coming to our home to help. Two caregivers told me after just a few appointments that they could not continue helping because of Jodie's reaction to them. The hopelessness of not having any solutions affected me greatly as I describe later in Section Seven: Caregiving from a Wheelchair. My search for solutions led to life-changing decisions that will be covered later in this book.

The next chapter describes how family, social and religious life can help you maintain a full and happy life despite your challenges.

---

* A description by the Cleveland Clinic can be found here. https://my.clevelandclinic.org/health/treatments/14330-male-sling-procedure

Acceptance and Adaptation

"None of us has the luxury of choosing our challenges; fate and history provide them for us.
Our job is to meet the tests we are presented."
—Jerome Powell, quoted in the *Wall Street Journal*,
April 27, 2020

This section on the acceptance of and adaptation to your changed circumstances contains three chapters. In the first, I describe how family, friends, and religion can help you lead a full life despite your medical challenges.

The second chapter focuses on maintaining your strength and the importance that can have in delaying the onset of new challenges, particularly if you have a progressive physical disease.

The third chapter suggests the kind of support network you will need to get things done that you used to do yourself.

3

Family, Social
and Religious Support

"It is not miracles that generate faith, but faith that generates miracles."
—Fyodor Dostoevsky, the voice of the narrator, describing the position of a realist, in *The Brothers Karamazov* (1880)

The support of your family, friends, church and religious beliefs are vital to helping you deal with your challenges. With this help, you can maintain a full and happy life. When I told my fraternity brother, Larry Haack, that I was writing a book to help others deal with the issues Jodie and I have faced, he said that his situation was similar to mine and added: "The issue of being physically limited is real and I survive with considerable assistance and support of my church."

My fraternity brother, Bob Lindsay, told me, "I have not found any useful support groups, but have benefited from talking with Dick Hamme* and others who are dealing with similar life hurdles.... Our faith community has been incredibly supporting and helpful."

Jodie and I have a great life and are very blessed. The most important reason for this is that we have a close, loving relationship that has lasted 53 years and counting. We express that to each other many times each day.

Almost as important is our extended family. We have great relationships with all of them. This includes our children, their spouses, our grandchildren, and other family members as well. My wife loves her cousins and we are both close to my extended family, which includes three siblings, their spouses, and their extended families. Since the early seventies, we have gotten together for a reunion every year. For decades this reunion has been for a full week. The reunions and other gatherings have helped all of us in many ways, including allowing our children and grandchildren to develop and maintain close relationships. Because we are all aware of the problems each of us is dealing with, we support each other emotionally and make suggestions for potential solutions. I have received many suggestions from all of my siblings and children that have helped me in my search for answers to our changing situations.

We also have many great friends living near us. Most of them were found

---

* Dick Hamme is another fraternity brother that is quoted in Chapter 26: Caregiving Introduction.

through Jodie's church. When we moved to California, she joined an aerobics group and became friends with several ladies. That led to social gatherings outside of aerobics. One of the girls invited Jodie to join a book club. Many of the girls in the book club were members of the same church and belonged to a church group called Renew, which Jodie joined. Renew met and still meets every Tuesday. They have a brief social discussion over coffee followed by a religious discussion for a couple of hours and then go to lunch for more social interaction. Jodie looks forward to each Tuesday's Renew and is well taken care of there. I know that the Renew group prays for both of us every week.

Soon after we moved to California, we joined a program Jodie's church offered called "Guess Who's Coming to Dinner," where couples were matched into groups each year. Each group's members rotated from home to home with the hostess preparing the main course and dessert and others bringing selected dishes. We became friends with George and Colleen Homolka, one of the couples from that program. Subsequently, Jodie invited Colleen to join the book club and Renew. Over time, we created a circle of great friends who got together in both large and small groups for other social occasions. We were close to Joel and Heather Elmore and Harold and Darleen Sochan. The wives were good friends and the men had a lot in common. Each of us had degrees in engineering, though in different fields. Unfortunately, as Jodie's and my circumstances changed, we couldn't participate in some of the social occasions that we used to attend, but this circle of friends greatly enhanced our lives.

Being so busy with work, I didn't develop many friends on my own. Fortunately, Jodie's closest friends had great husbands. While we were all working, I only saw George, Harold, and Joel when the couples got together. That changed after we all retired. Joel was the last to retire and was an avid golfer. He was the creator of our golf group, which became my primary social activity. We would play a round of golf and then go to lunch. Often, all four of us would play, but we would play at least once a week even if there were just two or three of us. Sometimes we would meet another time to go to the driving range to practice various parts of the game. Playing this much was new for me. It helped improve my game and made us all closer. Eventually, Harold and Darleen moved to Canada, their home country, which left us short one player. Subsequently, when Joel and I played as a twosome, we were joined by John Wyatt, who was playing as a single. He was a good fit in multiple ways so we invited him to join our group.

When I started showing signs of physical decline, I would still play golf but had to adjust to what I could do. I went from being one of the longest drivers in the group to the shortest to not able to hit a driver. What I did on the golf course reduced over time, dropping one club at a time until I ended up just chipping and putting. I had to drive a cart close to the green, get out of the cart and support myself with the four-legged cane and the handle of my club until I was ready to hit. One of my friends would take the cane and, after I hit, hand me the cane and the next club. If I had to go downhill to get on or off the green, someone would support me. My goal was to continue doing all I could until it was too dangerous. I have applied this philosophy to all my activities. Eventually, it became too risky to play golf, but I had the fun of playing and positive social interaction for a long time.

I was replaced in the golf group by Bill Swisher, another husband of one of Jodie's friends, but I still join the group for lunch. The lunch group has expanded to include Bob Totten, Terry's husband, yet another of Jodie's close friends. He doesn't play golf, but he has made these lunches even more enjoyable. At many of these lunches, my friends have offered valuable suggestions regarding how to solve the problems Jodie and I have faced.

We are also blessed to have some excellent neighbors. Steve and Jackie Steen have lived next door to us for more than 30 years. We have gone out to dinner as couples and Steve and I have had lunches together. When I was unable to drive, Steve offered to drive my SUV so the two of us could go to lunch or a movie. He has aided us in many ways. On the other side are Sara and Mark Ericson, who have also been very helpful. When they heard that my family was coming for Christmas, Mark and his daughter Anna came over and put Christmas lights out front. As you will see in subsequent chapters, our friends and neighbors have helped in numerous other ways.

I can't overemphasize the importance of having a good family, social and religious life. I encourage you to strengthen those ties and increase them to the extent possible. This will significantly improve the quality of your life.

One of the things you can only do yourself is to maintain or increase your physical strength as long as possible. This subject is covered in the next chapter.

4

Stay Healthy,
Maintain Your Strength

"Physical fitness is not only one of the most important keys to a healthy body, it is the basis of dynamic and creative intellectual activity."

—John F. Kennedy

When dealing with a progressive reduction in your strength, it is essential to do what you can to slow down that progression. Even if your condition isn't progressive, you need to maintain or increase your strength if you can. To get stronger, you have to break down muscle to build it. This seems counter-intuitive but is true. In a weightwatchers.com article by Leanna Carpenter titled "How Muscles Get Big,"[1] she quotes Michael Moses,* who explained: "When muscles are overloaded during weight lifting, little tears are made in the muscle itself. This microtrauma may sound harmful but is, in fact, the natural response of your muscles when they experience work. The muscle repairs these tears when you're resting, and this helps muscles grow in size and strength."

Before I noticed a decline in my strength, I had a recumbent bicycle machine in my home, and I went to the gym three or four times a week. Gymnasiums have many options for maintaining or improving your strength and conditioning.† I encourage you to find a gym near home or work, preferably one near restaurants, theaters, etc. In my case, I found one in a shopping center with restaurants, a theater, a grocery store, a bank, a hair salon, a medical center, etc. A picture of my wife Jodie and me enjoying Blackhawk Plaza is shown on the following page.

I am sitting on my walker as will be discussed in Chapter 7. This plaza provided an incentive for us to go to the gym even when we didn't feel like it. Jodie and I enjoyed the atmosphere and the quality of the restaurants and always took advantage of the things we could accomplish while there. At different times we saw a movie, bought groceries, got our hair cut, etc. When neither Jodie nor I could drive, this was even more important because we couldn't go anywhere

---

* Michael Moses, a team doctor for the Marine Corps Marathon, the Washington Football Team, the Washington Wizards, and others.

† A few examples for improving strength are the horizontal seated leg press, the lat pulldown, the cable biceps bar, the cable triceps bar, and the chest press. Examples for conditioning include elliptical machines, stair mills, spin bikes, recumbent bikes, and rowing machines.

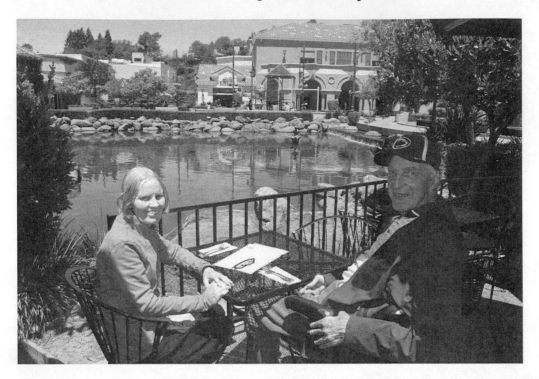

Enjoying Blackhawk Plaza (photograph by Mike Reed).

except via a Paratransit bus that could take me with my scooter. As a result, we got out only about once a week so it was important to accomplish multiple purposes when we could.

If you still have the capability of using the machines in your home or in a gymnasium, I highly recommend that you do it. It is vital to work out several times a week and continue as long as your doctor says it is safe. Maintaining your current condition as long as possible is well worth it and can delay the next challenges.

Many people find that having a trainer is a good idea because they know what you need, the best way to accomplish it, and will push you to go further than you would otherwise. Some people will also find that having an appointment with a trainer is a needed incentive to get to the gym.

One warning though, some trainers, particularly those who were college or pro athletes, can hurt you by pushing you too far. I once had a trainer who wanted to strengthen my ankles and calves by having me stand up on a platform supported only by the front of my feet. He asked me to rock up-and-down with my heels going above and below the platform. I told him that I had a surgically repaired ankle and was concerned about this exercise, but he said it would be fine.

Against my better judgment, I did the exercise and it ended up creating significant problems with my ankle, so I stopped using that trainer. You have to use your judgment; in that case, I didn't and suffered the consequences.

For various medical issues, many related to playing basketball, I've gone to a few physical therapists over the years. They know how far to push you and are better qualified to tell you what to do, what weights to use, and how many reps are appropriate. I would make a note of all the things that they specified. When my sessions were over, I would find the machines in the gym that would allow me to continue the recommended physical therapy routines. If you are disabled, your doctor can provide a prescription to see a physical therapist who can teach you what you need to do. Write down what exercises the physical therapist recommends and have the trainer work with you on those things. If you are highly self-motivated, you don't have to use a trainer; do these things on your own.

If you are 65 or older, check to see whether your insurance includes Silver Sneakers. If it does and there is a gym near you that accepts it, a gym membership is free. My insurance (Medicare with Blue Shield of California Supplemental) covered it for a while at my gym (Crunch) but later stopped. I assume Silver Sneakers negotiated a reduced rate, and the gym didn't need it for revenue or found it was reducing their income by members converting from paying customers to Silver Sneaker members. Many Medicare supplement and Medicare Advantage insurance plans include Silver Sneakers at no extra cost. If you have an AARP Silver Sneakers account (also known as United Healthcare Silver Sneakers), they may include Silver Sneakers, but they have stopped providing it in several states. Search for silversneakers.com where you can enter your insurance and location to see what is available to you.

For a long time, I was able to utilize the strength machines on my own. Eventually, I had to have someone lift the seat as high as possible on some of the machines to use them. I was too weak to do it myself. At least twice, I had terrible falls that brought the paramedics for a trip to the emergency room. This is the downside of pushing things too far. I took some unacceptable risks ... part of the learning process you want to avoid. Over time I realized that it was not safe to get off of the stair mill, then the elliptical machine, and then the treadmill. Eventually, to my great regret, I had to stop going to the gym because there was little I could do there.

After I dropped my gym membership, I had to find a way to keep exercising in the house. Because my mobility outside of the house was challenging, my doctor had an occupational therapist come to the house to evaluate me. Occupational therapists are highly specialized professionals who focus on the skill sets individuals require to function independently in the home or workplace.

She, in turn, sent a physical therapist, and he trained me how to do various exercises to maintain strength. I was surprised that my arms got a little bit stronger, which I didn't think was possible with my diseases. The therapist helped me identify what equipment I should buy that could be used in the house and provided a set of instructions for various exercises. It might not be necessary for you to have an occupational therapist come to your home, but you should get a referral to see one regardless. Medicare paid for it for me, and your insurance might do so as well. Exercises will be customized for your capabilities and targeted at those muscles that are most important.

There was one negative outcome with my home physical therapy. It was vital to build up the core of my body so that I could continue getting up out of my lift chair, scooter, etc. One of the exercises to accomplish this was to raise and hold my hips up in the air repeatedly while I was sitting in my lift chair. I had never done this exercise before, and unfortunately, after having done it several times, I got a severe muscle strain in my left inner thigh. I was in great pain when standing up, transferring from one piece of equipment to another, and taking off or putting on clothes. Jodie had to help me for some time. It made me almost completely immobile for many days.

Having had an experience earlier with a trainer harming me with an inappropriate exercise for my situation, you would think that I would have known better. However, I had no idea that this exercise would create such a problem. I learned from this that when you are getting physical therapy, do not let them over-stress you with any exercise you haven't done before or haven't done recently. Make sure they limit the number of reps initially and build them up over time in a conservative way. In my case, I had them stop that particular exercise completely. After completing all my sessions, I started bringing back that exercise very slowly because I knew it would be valuable as long as I didn't overdo it so much that it was counterproductive.

Even if you can maintain enough strength to accomplish certain things, you will need help from others to accomplish things you were once able to do yourself. The next chapter provides information on resources for the things you will likely need others to do for you.

5

Build Your Essential Help Network

*"The healthy, the strong individual, is the one who asks for help
when he needs it.
Whether he's got an abscess on his knee or in his soul."*
—Rona Barrett, in *Miss Rona: An Autobiography* (1977)

In Chapter 3, I discussed the importance of family, social and religious life and how they affect your quality of life and ability to cope emotionally with challenges. This chapter focuses on things you will need others to do for you. Frequent and infrequent issues will arise that need to be resolved quickly to improve your safety and comfort. For clarity, I have broken this chapter into several topics that outline what you will likely need.

Contractor

If you choose to continue living in your house, you will probably have to modify it. Through George from my golf group, I met Tim Heck, a contractor who can handle almost any construction project. Over the years, Tim has installed grab bars, replaced flooring, dealt with flood damage, repaired plumbing, installed an outside fountain, and many other things. His biggest project was to completely redo the master bathroom to accommodate my need to independently and safely shower. Finding a quality contractor like Tim who is available when needed and able to handle a broad scope of repairs and remodeling tasks is difficult but essential. Building a relationship with the contractor through multiple jobs and personal discussions is also important. As a result of doing this, I know that my contractor, on more than one occasion, moved us ahead of other clients when we needed something important done quickly.

Handyman

Many smaller tasks that you and your spouse used to be able to do will become difficult or impossible later. You will find that you need a handyman frequently, so you should find a competent and reliable handyman and foster that relationship. You may not find one person to do everything, but having relation-ships with people with the skills you need is vital. Our handyman, Tom Busta, can do almost anything. Over the years he has cleaned gutters, washed windows, helped us get ready for guests, organized things in the house, built shelving in the garage, done minor plumbing work, repaired doors damaged by my scooter, installed a ramp, cleaned out the garage when we got a second vehicle, and many other things. More recently, Tom built a platform and installed it under my lift chair to make it possible for me to continue to get up.

Gardener

I loved gardening but had to give it up; many of you will too. For many years we have used Javier Arias, an excellent gardener. He and his family members come once a week and do the usual things like mowing, weeding, and trimming bushes. I also use him on special projects, e.g., picking up an order of flowers at a nursery and planting them. Once a year Javier trims trees. About twice a year he sprays the base of the house to prevent ants from gaining entry. He has dug French drains to help with drainage and sold us firewood. He does a great job and is very pleasant. If you find a good one, incentivize him to stay. I found that the extra projects helped accomplish that for me.

House Cleaner

This used to be a shared responsibility in our home but now neither of us can do very much. I have significant limitations and Jodie's condition eliminates almost everything she used to do. You may find you can't do all you need to do either. It took a while, but we found Maria Javier, a cleaning lady who is more thorough than any other we have used. She is also reliable and trustworthy. We are comfortable not being in the house when she is there. This relieves Jodie of that responsibility and allows us to be better prepared for guests. Initially, we scheduled her as needed, but now we have her clean on a regular schedule. Put-ting her on a regular schedule helped us keep this valuable resource.

Help from Family, Friends and Neighbors

If you are fortunate enough to have family living nearby, you may get a lot of assistance from them. Unfortunately, that is not the case for us. All children, grandchildren, and siblings live states away, most on the opposite coast. Many of your friends and neighbors are likely to offer to help. I accept some offers but not if I think it is too much of an imposition. An example of this is when Steve, my neighbor and friend, volunteered to drive me to Sacramento, California, which is more than an hour and a half away. I needed to be evaluated by a Certified

Driver Rehabilitation Specialist (CDRS®).* It was a critical meeting to see whether I could safely drive with hand controls, and would involve most of the day. I turned Steve down because I didn't believe it was appropriate to ask so much of a neighbor and instead asked my son to fly up from Phoenix to take me.

There are instances when it is necessary to accept or even ask for help. However, I believe independence is the goal and imposing on others should be minimized. Help should be requested only when you don't have a reasonable alternative and know your request will be positively received. I use gift cards and inviting people out to dinner to show my appreciation. When I had a water leak, I called Steve and he rushed over to shut off the water in the middle of the night. He has responded to my home alarm when it went off by mistake. When I found I needed to raise my bed, I purchased some bed risers and he came over to install them. When the battery in my motor scooter was dying and I was unable to open up the battery pack to replace the batteries, he did that for me.

I asked for help when I needed to make two trips to another town to determine which vehicle would work best for driving with my wheelchair. To minimize the burden on one individual, I asked Steve to take me on one trip and my golf group friend, John, for the other. John drives me to lunch every week and I knew both Steve and John would be happy to help. Joel, another golf partner, always calls me before he goes to Costco and certain restaurants and asks for a list of things to pick up.

Some of Jodie's friends have offered to acquire food or other things for us, as have my neighbors Steve and Sara. So far I have not taken them up on any of those kind offers because I want to be as independent as possible and I don't want to lean on other people too much. However, it is nice to have people who want to help you when you need it.

To illustrate my neighbors' helpfulness, I will relate a problem with a power outage in the early evening. Both Steve and Sara called to find out whether we had eaten dinner. Sara's husband Mark was cooking on a camp stove and offered to cook something for us. Both neighbors knew that I would not be able to get to the bedroom or bathroom if the outage extended long enough because I would have to use an electric lift to get to that level of the house. Steve offered to come over and try the hand crank backup system and Sara and Mark offered to bring over a portable generator when I wanted to go to bed if the power was still out. Fortunately, the power came on but it is great to have neighbors so willing to help without even being asked.

Help from Fraternity Brothers

This category is a late addition to the book, but it would be remiss not to include my fraternity brothers because they made many significant contributions to this book.

---

* There is a chapter later in this book about Certified Driver Rehabilitation Specialists.

After college, I was so consumed with family and career that I lost track of my Triangle fraternity brothers at Penn State. Fred Bowman, a roommate in college, was the exception. Fred and I never lost touch. As a consultant, I functioned as Chief Operating Officer for one of his medical instrument companies for a while.

We agreed that it was regrettable that we lost contact with our brothers and resolved to correct this. I found Dave Cowles on Facebook and the three of us networked to find more brothers. Once Harlan Byers became a member, he helped us rapidly expand the membership until we had more than 40 members in our group from the years we were together. We created an online album where we posted old photos of our house and parties and updated pictures of ourselves and our families. That was shocking! We created an online document where we shared stories of our time at Penn State and provided updates on our families' lives and our careers.

The group was formed in late 2017, long before I had any thought of writing a book. When I notified the group of my intent and told them the book's scope, I got considerable encouragement and help from my brothers.

Many of them or their wives had faced difficulties of their own. They freely described their challenges and how they dealt with them, hoping to help others. Multiple quotes from them are included in this book.

Fred Hellrich helped me in multiple ways. He reviewed those chapters where he had information that would be helpful and offered suggestions. Fred provided significant content for one chapter. When I faced a challenging, short-term move, he suggested an organization that would be helpful. Through that tip, I found someone who was crucial in accomplishing the move to a senior living facility in Arizona on time. He also suggested a way to self-publish if I had trouble finding a publisher.

Conclusion

Having a way to quickly and effectively get things done is essential. If you don't have this type of support, you should do all you can to get it.

The next section of this book describes the best ways to ensure your personal mobility, one of the most important capabilities required to ensure your quality of life. It starts with initial solutions that are effective in the early stages of a progressive disease. Subsequent chapters cover the devices you may need as you become more debilitated.

Safe Personal Mobility Solutions

"Those who overcome great challenges will be changed, and often in unexpected ways.
For our struggles enter our lives as unwelcome guests, but they bring valuable gifts.
And once the pain subsides, the gifts remain.
These gifts are life's true treasures, bought at great price, but cannot be acquired in any other way."

—Steve Goodier

Personal mobility is one of the most important functions needed to maintain your quality of life. Your mobility and the equipment you need will change as your disease progresses. In this section, I share my experience, the decisions I made, and why I made them. I also provide information to allow you to make different decisions if your situation and goals differ from mine.

Getting insurance coverage for medical equipment can be very challenging. However, I have been successful in getting what I wanted using the procedure provided below. It took a very frustrating and time-consuming effort to get approval for my wheelchair, described in Chapter 9. I found that some doctors aren't aware of which Medicare codes will be approved. The amount of coordination required between the equipment supplier, the occupational therapist (OT), and the doctors can be extraordinary.

The recommended procedure follows:

1. Decide what equipment you think you need, e.g., a motorized wheelchair.
2. Do some personal research on the brands and models available and the features that you think you need.
3. Visit an Abilities Expo or an equipment dealer to try out the equipment and discuss the pros and cons of the available models and features with the dealer.
4. Get a referral from your neurologist to an OT.

5. Explain in detail to the OT why you need the specific manufacturer, model, and each of the features you want. Ensure that your explanation of why you need the equipment and the features requested is based entirely on in-home use because Medicare doesn't cover needs outside the home.
6. Coordinate the manufacturer's efforts and the OT to create a document for the neurologist, including an appropriate Medicare code. I have provided a list in Chapter 9 that should work. Review it before it is sent to the neurologist. The neurologist will most likely use that document, or the information in it, in their submittal to the insurance entity, significantly increasing your odds of getting insurance coverage for exactly what you want.
7. Ensure your neurologist includes a code in the submittal that will be approved, specifying the medical condition that makes this equipment necessary. I found that some GPs and neurologists enter codes that will not be approved. I suggest that you show them the list I have provided and encourage them to use the closest applicable code to your condition.

This procedure reflects one of the themes of this book.... *Be your own advocate.*

6

Initial Solutions

"When everything seems to be going against you, remember that the airplane takes off against the wind, not with it."

—Henry Ford

When it comes to mobility equipment, the natural tendency is to delay the decision to acquire something safer, whether moving from a cane to a walker or from a motorized scooter to a motorized wheelchair. Some of the reasons for this reluctance include vanity, loss of a sense of independence, inconvenience, cost, and denial of the risk you are taking. However, there can be significant consequences when delaying these decisions.

My friend John Wyatt told me about a relative of his wife who had suffered a physical decline. He also cared for his wife, who was suffering from mental decline. John thought it would be beneficial for me to meet him for my own sake and for some insight that would be helpful for my book. Before setting the meeting time, I learned that the man fell and died of a head injury. He had been using only a cane and had not acquired a safer mobility device. This is an extreme example, but it may encourage you to make decisions on safer mobility devices sooner. After John's relative's experience, and my falls, some of which had resulted in going to the emergency room with injuries, my approach changed.

I developed a great fear of catastrophic falls, especially when walking outside on a hard surface. Nightmares resulted in which I was falling. I would swing my arms to save myself and slam my hand into the headboard. After deciding I needed a cane, I bought a collapsible single-leg one. It worked for a while, as I learned how to quickly poke around in the appropriate direction to prevent falls.

Later feeling I needed something safer, I considered a HurryCane* or a four-legged cane. I chose to acquire a four-legged cane that had a larger footprint. The collapsible single-leg cane was more convenient on trips, but in retrospect, I should have gone directly to the four-legged one. I used the four-legged cane for quite a while, but the fear and the nightmares remained. On the following page is a picture of the canes I used.

Because my falls were caused by my left leg collapsing, I sought a solution to that particular problem. The collapses seemed to be caused by a momentary loss

---

* Search HurryCane on the Internet for available models.

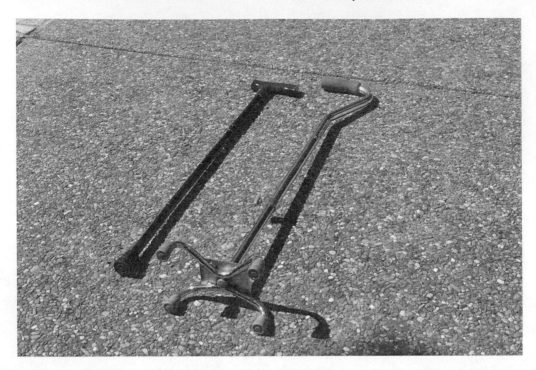

One-legged and four-legged canes I used (photograph by the author).

of signal from the brain to the muscle when taking a step. There were occasions when I had resisted falling by grabbing onto something as the fall started. Then, after a brief moment, the leg worked normally. As I had an engineering education, I thought there should be equipment available to resist a sudden collapse long enough to avoid a fall caused by a momentary lack of muscle response. A similar principle was used in the moveable concrete barriers for highways sold by Barrier Systems Inc. (BSI)[*] of which I was a part-owner and director for many years. After I discussed this with my neurologist, she sent me to an occupational therapist. The therapist told me that they could make a leg brace that would be helpful, but what I wanted was available only for prosthetics, not for orthotics.[†] War casualties and accidents have created a large need for this capability for prosthetics, but there is an insufficient market for that type of function for orthotics.

I used the procedure outlined in the introduction of this section to get approval for the orthotic; it was approved. A brace was fitted for me and is pictured on the next page.

However, the brace couldn't resist the collapse without locking up, which is what I needed. The brace was designed to lock up, much like a seat belt in a car accident. That could work at times, but I was worried about what would happen if I fell anyway. Fearing that a locked leg could cause even more damage because I

---

[*] There are permanent applications of these barriers on highways and bridges, e.g., the Golden Gate Bridge. They are also used temporarily in construction zones. Search "Barrier Systems Inc." for more information.

[†] Orthotics enhance the function of a limb while prosthetics are used to replace a missing limb.

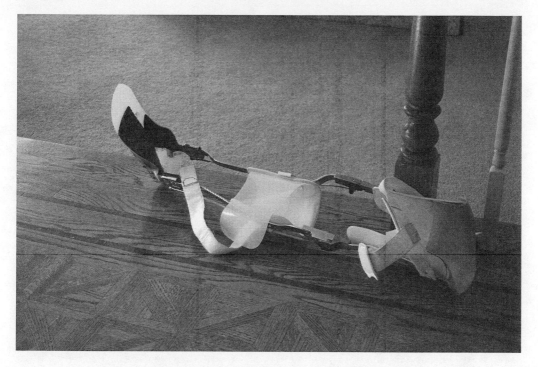

Leg brace I tried (photograph by the author).

couldn't move my leg during a fall, I abandoned its use. Other orthotics might be an option for your needs, however.

Once I determined that the canes and the leg brace were no longer safe, it was time to find a better mobility device. The next chapter explains what I chose and why.

7

Rolling Walker

"You have to look at yourself objectively. Analyze yourself like an instrument.
You have to be absolutely frank with yourself. Face your handicaps, don't try to hide them...."

—Audrey Hepburn

Deciding that the leg brace and the canes were unsafe, I looked for another solution. A walker seemed the best answer. There are standard walkers and rolling walkers (walkers with wheels). I didn't consider a standard walker. While they are more stable than a rolling walker, I don't recommend them for people who have a progressive disease. You have to lift them to move. The user has to have good upper body strength, but that is often not the case. Also, it takes longer when using one to get where you are going. However, they might be suitable for your situation. If you choose to use a standard walker, you can try cutting tennis balls and putting them on the legs to enable you to slide the walker across many surfaces.

There are many variations of rolling walkers. They can have two, three, or four wheels. Another name for a four-wheel rolling walker is a rollator. For this book, I will use the generic term "rolling walker" or "walker." The wheels can be large or small. It is important to find the walker suitable for your size and condition. I have seen many people with a walker that didn't look stable enough for their condition or was not properly sized. I have also seen people bent way over because the handles were too low; that can create back problems. I chose a four-wheel walker with large wheels because of the stability and ease of walking. Cost and other considerations might lead you to a different decision.

Whatever decision you make, be sure your walker fits you and your situation well. There are guides for choosing the right walker. A good website for this is the Mayo Clinic.[*] They describe the types of walkers, how to choose a grip, how to get the right size, and other useful information. Another website with this type of information is justwalkers.com.[†] The specific web address in the footnote provides additional valuable information. For example, one link on that page titled "How to Measure for a Walker" describes how to choose a walker's size, which is

---

[*] Search "Mayo Clinic: Tips for Choosing a Walker"
[†] https://justwalkers.com/pages/walkers-tips.

similar to how my occupational therapist sized mine. She had me stand by the walker with my shoes on. With my arms down by my side, she measured the distance from my wrist to the floor. This is the ideal height from the floor to the walker's handles, but your walker should have some ability to adjust the height to suit you.

I can attest to the importance of proper height. I avoided many incipient falls by pushing straight down on the walker's handles when my legs failed me momentarily. A fall I had in Costco demonstrates why being able to push straight down is important. Believing I would have enough support by using the Costco cart's handles, I chose not to use my walker, which would have required a Costco employee to accompany me with the shopping cart.* A very serious fall resulted, two bruised knees, a sprained wrist and a sprained ankle. That night I couldn't get up from my chair because of the sprained wrist. I realized that when my legs started to collapse, I could not push down because my arms were out in front of me, and the handles were too high. Even with a walker, this could happen if the arms of your walker were too high or you were standing too far back from the handles.

The width of the walker is another consideration. Make sure that you'll be able to go through your home and into commercial bathroom stalls before you purchase.

As I mentioned earlier, my solution was a four-wheel rolling walker with a seat. I chose Nova GetGo. It had the highest seat and highest handles, which would help me get up from the walker seat when I was sitting on it. Being able to sit on the walker seat was another advantage of the GetGo.

I met some resistance in getting the make and model I needed but was ultimately successful using the process explained in the introduction to Section Three. An important part of that process was to explain in detail to the OT what my needs were, why I needed a four-wheel rolling walker, why the seat and handles had to be high, why I needed brakes,† and why the Nova GetGo was the answer. I asked that my needs be included in the OT's report to the neurologist. Once a supplier was chosen, I had to communicate with them a few times before I was provided with what met my needs. Originally, they intended to supply a walker that wasn't suitable. I got the walker in late December 2014 or January 2015. It would be my mobility device for almost two years and remains useful today.

Throughout this book, a message you will see and can't be overemphasized is that you have to be your own advocate. You need to make sure the right paperwork and insurance codes are supplied to the insurance provider, that the vendor fully understands your needs, and then be insistent on getting what you need from the vendor to ensure success.

---

* Most stores will provide a "personal shopper" when requested by a handicapped customer.

† Brakes are required on a rolling walker to limit speed on downslopes. Squeezing the lever under the handles applies the brakes. When you don't want the walker to move the brakes can be locked by pushing the levers down. This is helpful when transferring to or from the walker or getting up from the walker seat.

The GetGo has a large storage area under the seat which is very useful. It would also fold up so I could put it in the back seat when I was driving.

Pictured below is my rolling walker.

Once I started using the walker, my falls almost completely stopped. Even though I had one-step level changes in the house and a two-step change to the garage, I was able to safely manage that with the walker. The walker was and continues to be a great decision. It prevented falls and nightmares immediately. Initially, I used it only while walking outdoors. Later, I sat on it at restaurants because of its high seat, as shown in the first picture in the book, and at home when I couldn't get up from chairs. I used it to get to the shower because, at that time, I had to step over a curb height threshold to get in.

In subsequent chapters, I explain that my mobility device later became a motorized scooter and then a motorized wheelchair. My toilet/shower room was modified and I bought a specialized toilet/shower chair. Through all those changes, the rolling walker was and is in use daily. I place it beside my bed and use it as a transfer device to and from the bed and the mobility device. Another reason for having the walker beside my bed is that I get up to urinate about three times a night. To reduce the time to accomplish this, the stress on my muscles, and the ability to return to sleep sooner, I keep a male urinal on the walker's seat. With its high handles, the walker helps me steady myself when I get up. It is then unnecessary to get up, transfer to the scooter or wheelchair, go to the bathroom, get up onto my commode and then reverse the process to get to bed. A side benefit of having the walker beside the bed is the large storage area under the seat. I keep

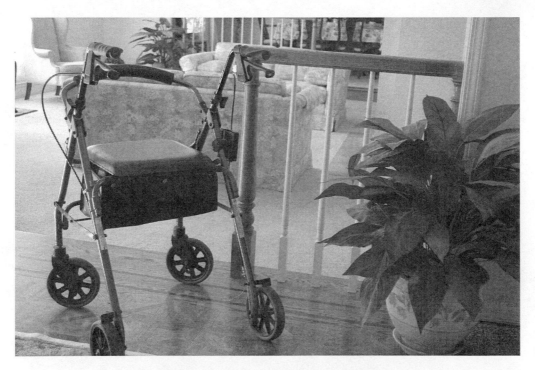

Rolling walker or rollator (photograph by the author).

items I might need while in bed and other necessities in that compartment, e.g., a flashlight, alarm clock, TV controller, reading glasses, etc.

This cane to walker progression is a case where I didn't think far enough ahead. Ego and convenience had caused me to delay the decision to acquire the walker. A better decision would have been to get the walker and a four-legged cane right away. I might not have wanted to take the walker on plane trips early on, but I could have used the four-legged cane on those trips.

While the walker lasted almost two years as my mobility device and was very safe during that period, having a progressive disease makes things that are safe at one time no longer safe at another. Progressive disease obviates old solutions. Again my muscles deteriorated; I needed something better than the walker. Down slopes, even handicap ramps posed the real threat of my knee collapsing. The walker could not save me in that type of situation.

Once I found myself in a situation where I had to go down a steep slope. I froze for quite a while. The same fear of falls I had previously experienced returned. The concern about a potential fall was magnified by the fact that I have osteoporosis. I suffered bruised ribs, a broken toe, sprains, and bruises from prior falls, and a broken hip and other potential injuries would have prevented me from having any mobility for a long time. I got out of that situation with my wife's help but knew I needed yet another solution.

If you face a similar need for mobility, a manual wheelchair might be a solution. This would be suitable only if you were able to get up from it, were strong enough to move it up slopes or always had someone to help you. That wasn't the case for me. I needed something motorized. In the next chapter, I describe and evaluate the pros and cons of motorized mobility options.

8

Motorized Scooter

*"What we eventually accomplish may depend more on our passion
and perseverance than on our innate talent."*
—Angela Duckworth, *Grit: The Power of Passion
and Perseverance*

When the walker was no longer safe, the choices for a motorized mobility device were a scooter and a wheelchair. There are significant advantages and disadvantages of each device so the decision might not be obvious. For this reason, I will start with a summary of each device's pros and cons, a subject I know well because I have experienced both. Table 1 provides an overview of the decision factors listed in order of importance and which device has the advantage in each case.

This chapter explains why I chose a scooter as my first mobility device, which scooter I bought, why I chose it, and how I used and maintained it. Finally, I discuss why the scooter was useful even after my physical progression made it clear that it could no longer be my primary mobility device.

Table 1 shows which device has the advantage for each factor but doesn't explain how I made those evaluations. The following list provides information on how I made those evaluations for these essential decision-making factors. I have listed them in order of my assessment of their importance. Your priorities could differ from mine, but this list should help you decide whether a walker or wheelchair best meets your needs.

Standing and Transferring: Substantial Advantage Wheelchair

There are many situations where you want or need to stand briefly if you can do so. At other times, you have to stand to transfer to another device. It is much easier and much safer to stand and transfer from a wheelchair because the seat is higher. Also, you can tilt the seat and get an elevation option making the wheelchair even more advantageous. However, in tight quarters where you have to transfer at a 90-degree angle, the scooter is better because you can turn its seat to stand or transfer. It's not possible to turn the seat in a wheelchair and there often isn't sufficient room to turn the entire wheelchair. I assigned the highest priority to this need, as standing and transferring occurs frequently and can be dangerous. Struggling to stand can also tire your muscles, making it difficult to transfer late in the day.

	SCOOTER	WHEELCHAIR
Standing and Transferring		Substantial Advantage
Access to Rooms	Substantial Advantage	
Transporting Objects	Substantial Advantage	
Access to Elevated Levels		Substantial Advantage
Getting Close	Substantial Advantage	
Travel Distance		Substantial Advantage
Comfort and Pressure Sores		Substantial Advantage
Maneuvering in the Home		Advantage
Safety	Advantage	
Capital Cost	Advantage	
Maintenance Cost	Advantage	
Convenience	Advantage	

Table 1: Scooter vs. Wheelchair Comparison.

Access to Rooms: Substantial Advantage Scooter

Scooters are relatively narrow and can get through smaller spaces. Wheelchairs are wider and many doors in a typical house are too narrow to accommodate them. If you choose a wheelchair, this access problem will force you to make life-changing decisions. If you stay in your home, you will either lose access to some rooms or have to widen the doors at a high cost. If you leave, you must find another place to live that can accommodate a wheelchair. That raises social, financial and tax issues that will be discussed later. I ranked this factor second because of the impact it can have on your life.

Transporting Objects: Substantial Advantage Scooter

The scooter has a front basket and a floor that can be used to transport items. It also has a pouch on the backside of the seat. You can even add a large basket on the back. These features allow you to do much that you are unable to do with a walker or wheelchair. Examples include taking out the trash; doing laundry; taking food and drinks to the kitchen table or your lift chair and carrying sunglasses, keys, cell phones, wallets, eyeglasses, garage door openers, etc. The wheelchair cannot transport anything and that's a big problem. I rated this factor third because of its impact on your daily life and independence.

Access to Elevated Levels: Substantial Advantage Wheelchair

There is much that can't be reached from a scooter. This will mean that you aren't as independent as you would like because you will need help. Also, you are then tempted to stand to accomplish these tasks, particularly when no one is available to help, which is very risky. Wheelchairs are taller and you can get an elevation option, making it is possible to reach into cabinets, the freezer, etc. I rated this factor fourth because of its impact on your independence.

Getting Close: Substantial Advantage Scooter

It is important to be able to get close to things like chairs, tables, and sinks. Coming in parallel to the item with the scooter and turning the seat 90 degrees allows you to do this easily. This helps you get ready for the day at your sink, get close to a restaurant table, and similar situations. The wheelchair needs to be right in front of the chair, sink, etc. There is also the danger of injuring your feet which stick out in front of the wheelchair. It is hard to reach what you need with a wheelchair. You can come in at an angle but have to turn your body, which can create stress. I ranked this factor fifth because the need to get close to things occurs throughout the day and because of injury potential when using the wheelchair.

Travel Distance: Substantial Advantage Wheelchair

Relative to a wheelchair, a scooter has a limited range. That range declines as the battery weakens and it is possible to get stranded. Wheelchair batteries are designed so that the wheelchair can go long distances, well beyond a scooter.

Comfort and Pressure Sores: Substantial Advantage Wheelchair

Wheelchairs are fitted to your body and various types of cushioned seats are available. In addition, wheelchairs have various important capabilities like tilting and reclining, allowing you to change and spread your weight over larger surfaces. This helps avoid pressure sores, which can create serious medical problems. Scooters have none of these capabilities. I ranked this factor seventh, but the rating is heavily dependent upon the length of time you expect to be in your mobility device daily. This relatively low rating applies if you don't expect to be in the mobility device many hours a day, especially if you spend significant time in a lift chair where you can shift your weight frequently. The rating would be much higher if you were confined to a mobility device most of the day.

Maneuvering in the Home: Advantage Wheelchair

As explained earlier, a scooter can get through narrow doors when a wheelchair can't, so it ranked higher regarding access to rooms. However, maneuvering in a home often requires multiple back and forth movements to get where you want to with a scooter. With a wheelchair, you can more quickly go wherever you want in one move because of the tighter turning radius of wheelchairs. This is particularly true with mid-wheel drive wheelchairs. However, there is an important drawback to a wheelchair when moving through long narrow spaces like entering a lift. As explained in the next chapter, it is much more difficult to keep a wheelchair moving straight through in these situations if you have to reverse direction. I assigned the advantage to the wheelchair because most homes don't have lifts or similar adaptations for these situations.

Safety: Advantage Scooter

In the paragraph on getting close to things, I mentioned that your feet stick out in front of a wheelchair. This can cause minor injuries if you aren't constantly vigilant. In a scooter, your feet are well protected on a platform behind the front of the scooter and steering column, thus that injury isn't possible. Each device has the potential for dangerous unintended movement which can cause injury or damage. Why this can happen with a scooter and how to avoid it is described later in this chapter. A wheelchair can cause a similar problem. How it can happen and ways to minimize the risk are discussed in the next chapter. The wheelchair has more safety concerns resulting in my awarding the scooter the advantage.

Capital Cost: Advantage Scooter

The scooter is much cheaper if you have to pay for your mobility device yourself, as I did with the scooter for reasons explained later. However, my wheelchair would have been fully covered if I hadn't added the elevation option.

Maintenance Cost: Advantage Scooter

The wheelchair has more useful features but they are electronic, so more things can go wrong. However, after one year your health care insurance pays for maintenance costs, in my case Medicare and supplemental insurance. Also, it is unusual for a significant maintenance cost to occur in the first year.

Convenience: Advantage Scooter

Many scooters are convenient for travel in a commercial airline because they can be taken apart and folded down. If your wheelchair has a sealed gel-cell battery, there is no chance of chemicals spilling so they are allowed on airplanes as well. Scooters often have a headlight, which you only get with an expensive light package for a wheelchair.

Decision Rationale

For my condition and situation when the walker was no longer safe, the scooter was the obvious choice. By choosing the scooter:

1. I could access all the rooms in the house and I didn't have to face a life-altering decision to leave our home or pay for significant modifications to widen the doors.
2. I could transport things that enabled me to do the laundry, take out the trash, etc.

3. I could get close to things because the scooter seat can rotate to multiple positions.
4. It would be easier to get on the lifts in my house because they are barely wide enough for a wheelchair but have good clearance for the scooter.
5. The capital cost would be much less. (At that time, I only needed a mobility device outside the home so Medicare wouldn't cover a scooter or a wheelchair.)
6. There would be no risk of damaging my feet.
7. There would be minimal maintenance costs and no insurance was required.
8. It would be easier to travel by plane and my scooter would have a headlight.

The decision to get a scooter involved compromises relative to a wheelchair but they weren't as significant or critical as the scooter's positives at that time. There were additional facts that supported the scooter decision:

1. At the time of the decision, I could still stand and transfer to all necessary locations, so the wheelchair advantage was minimal. Because you can't turn the wheelchair seat at right angles and its size, it would negatively affect how I would use the toilet and a shower chair.
2. If I were not able to transport things my wife, Jodie, and I would be affected greatly. In her condition, doing things like the laundry and taking out the trash would be impossible without constant directions from me, many of which would not be understood. This would create great stress and conflict. The scooter decision eliminated this concern.
3. I found ways to deal with being unable to reach things at high levels. Jodie helped a lot and I had my handyman reorganize shelves and closets so I could reach what was most important. The most significant solution was how I handled dishes. After running the dishwasher, I would leave all the clean dishes in the dishwasher within easy reach. Dirty dishes were put in a deep sink. When the dishwasher was nearly empty, the rest of the clean dishes were moved to a drying rack on the counter and the dirty dishes were put in the dishwasher and washed. With these changes, the need for elevation was minimized.
4. By keeping the battery charged, monitoring the battery while traveling, and changing the batteries when necessary, the scooter travel distance was acceptable.
5. I wasn't going to spend many hours in the scooter a day and spent more hours in a lift chair where I could shift my weight frequently, so I didn't judge pressure sores as a significant risk.
6. For plane trips, my scooter seat can be removed by simply pulling it up. Once the seat is removed, the battery pack can also be removed by pulling it up. Then the steering column can be folded down onto the platform. The backrest folds down onto the removed seat area. In addition, at the end of the trip, the scooter can be driven and put into an ordinary car.

Airline travel with a motorized wheelchair is more problematic because you need a vehicle that can transport the wheelchair when you reach your destination. Thus, airline travel is more convenient with a scooter.

As stated earlier, after considering all these factors, I was confident the scooter was the right choice for me at that time. Still, there were also other considerations beyond just a comparison of pros and cons compared to a wheelchair. For example, I was still driving and knew I could transport the scooter with my SUV on a motorized platform on the back. The section on vehicle mobility will address how that was accomplished. Even after I couldn't drive, I knew that others could drive the SUV and transport the scooter and me. With a wheelchair, I would need an expensive, specially-modified van.

Another factor supporting the scooter decision was it would be useful even after I had a wheelchair. Given that I had progressive disease, I correctly assumed that I would eventually need a wheelchair, but I realized that the scooter's advantages would still be significant. I could use it to serve as a backup if the wheelchair were being serviced. Because some tasks are much easier to perform with the scooter, I could use it to take out the trash and do laundry one day a week. Until the doors were widened in the house, I would have access to rooms not accessible with the wheelchair. Yet another possible user was Jodie. She sometimes had trouble with long walks due to back pain, uncomfortable shoes or fatigue. We love getting out to take a "walk." Having both the scooter and the wheelchair would significantly extend the ability to do this because she could drive the scooter while I drove the wheelchair.

After performing my evaluation, I chose the Pride Go-Go Sport 4-Wheel scooter because of its stability and height. For me, it was much easier to get up from that model relative to other models from Pride or other manufacturers. I paid a local medical equipment dealer $1,953 for the scooter. I am pictured with my scooter on the next page.

As mentioned previously, the scooter gave me the ability to accomplish chores that I had not been able to do, e.g., laundry and trash. More important than those weekly uses for transporting things were the hourly ones. When I could no longer get up from the chair in my office or get to places in that room, I effectively lost the ability to use the office. The lift chair, and that which is surrounding it, e.g., the raised hearth of the fireplace and a tray, became my office. Getting up and transferring to get materials or to take them away and then reversing the process was tiring to my muscles. Tired muscles made going to bed more challenging and, at times, required Jodie's assistance. The scooter's basket and platform made it possible for me to reduce the number of trips significantly. Now I could carry much more at a time.

Some special options can be purchased with a scooter. One of them is a larger basket that hangs off the back of the chair. It is easy to install and remove. You just pull out a pin to remove it and replace the pin to put it back on. I purchased one and used it for a time. It was useful for carrying bags out of the grocery store but there was a significant drawback. When going into some elevators, I could barely

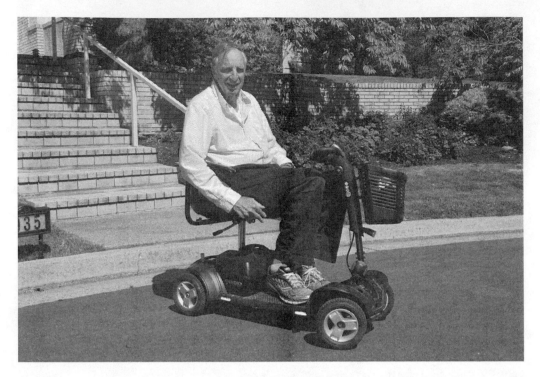

On my Pride Go-Go Sport Scooter (photograph by Taylor Bland).

fit because the basket hung off the back. Also, I would occasionally back into things or hit things when I turned, so eventually, I stopped using it. I also bought a cup holder so that I could carry a beverage. I don't advise buying it. I only used mine for a couple of weeks before it got knocked off when I moved through a narrow area outside. I didn't think it was important enough to buy another. However, you may find these options valuable.

The Go-Go Sport comes with a battery pack that has two internal batteries. Over time the batteries age and your travel distance will diminish. This is something you have to watch carefully. If you don't keep track of what's happening with your batteries, you may find yourself stranded. The battery indicator doesn't help much because the lights showing battery strength are not accurate. Even if all lights are on indicating full battery strength, there might be little battery strength left. While you are on ground level or going downhill, the lights can be all lit up, but as you go up a slope, they can quickly disappear. Once I had to have someone push me up the hill on my street and then up my driveway. My neighbor and wife have had to push a few times as well. In all of those cases, I had easily gone the same route and distance earlier. The best way to monitor the battery strength is to watch how many lights go out on up slopes. If you push it too much, the scooter will shut down. This happened once when I was at a one-week reunion, a long way from home. Fortunately, there is a reset button. You need to know where that is. On my scooter, it is on the front of the battery pack and is covered in a little plastic case.

In October 2017, I bought a backup charger from SpinLife for $109. I realized that I couldn't go anywhere, even in the house, without the scooter so I needed to have charged batteries. I can't walk at all and, while I can use a walker to perform transfers, it would be very unsafe to try to walk any distance with the walker. In January 2018, I also bought a backup battery pack from Amazon for $300 for the same reason. I recommend that you do the same if you have similar mobility issues.

Each battery pack has two internal batteries. My scooter uses two 16Ah internal batteries. My battery packs significantly weakened over time, and I could not travel to a local park anymore. It is possible to remove screws from the battery pack casing and lift out the internal batteries. I found a video on YouTube to watch the process. I decided to replace the batteries in only one of the battery packs and keep the other battery pack charged. It could still be used for short trips and would be a backup if something went wrong with the main battery pack. I bought replacement internal batteries in May 2019 from Amazon for $73 and my neighbor replaced the internal batteries in the weakest battery pack. Once I replaced the internal batteries, my distance capability greatly increased, allowing us to safely reach the park.

The manufacturer recommends that you charge the batteries only once a day (typically at night) for 8 to 10 hours. You should not charge for short periods for longer battery life, nor should you keep the charger connected after the batteries are fully charged. I found that I couldn't follow these recommendations entirely because I never knew when Jodie might want to go for a long walk. If I didn't have a fully charged battery pack ready, I would be uncertain about how far we could go. If there were any chance we might want to take a long walk, I would fully charge the battery during the day.

The decision to use the scooter in the house forced the decision to either move to another home with no level changes or purchase lifts and/or ramps. We love our house and grounds and have excellent views from the house. We live in a great location and have good friends nearby as well, so moving wasn't an attractive option. A ramp would work from the family room to the back patio, but we needed to add three lifts inside the house. Considering all the positives of staying in the home, we purchased the lifts and ramps. The chapter on house level changes provides more information on this subject.

Over time I found that getting up from the scooter became more difficult and a little more dangerous. This was because the braking system uses the inertia of the single motor that drives the scooter to keep it from moving. Sometimes that isn't sufficient given the force I had to put on the scooter to get up.

I bought some truck chocks that I could put behind and in front of a wheel to prevent movement. However, when I started to use a specialized toilet/shower chair, I couldn't use chocks. After I got up from a scooter to the toilet, I had to move the scooter back out of the shower room to maneuver to the shower, and chocks would prevent that. The chapter on showering safely provides more details on how I solved this problem. I have found through this journey that there exist workable solutions to the issues as they arise.

The scooter's directional movement is controlled by a one-piece toggle switch that sticks out from the steering column on both the right and left sides. The toggle is pinned in the middle so if it is pulled backward on the right it will move forward on the left. This makes it possible to control both forward and backward movement with either hand which can be useful at times. To avoid confusion, I recommend that you pull back on the toggle's right side to go forward and pull back on the left to go backward. To make sure this is clear, I have shown two pictures below. The first shows the neutral position when at rest. The second shows the forward position, but to show more of the toggle, I have moved my hands out of the picture as far as possible and pushed forward on the left side of the toggle.

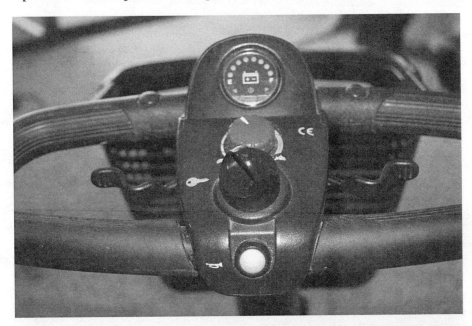

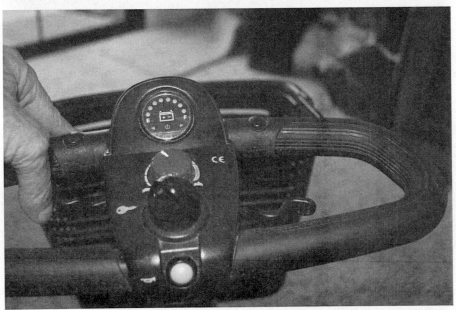

Speed is controlled in two ways. The circular knob shown in the pictures above between the key and the battery indicator works like a governor or speed limiter. The white line on the knob is at 11 o'clock in the picture, which would limit the speed to a moderate level. Rotating the knob fully clockwise would allow the maximum speed possible. Limiting the speed can minimize problems by avoiding sudden lurches that could be problematic. I always turn the knob to about 9 o'clock when someone new uses it for the first time. The extent to which you pull back on the toggle allows fine control of speed. Slight movement results in slower speed. Pulling it back all the way increases the speed to that permitted by the governor. It helps set the governor to the speed you want for long-distance travel because it is less stressful to pull the toggle back against the stop.

However, I found that there is a risk associated with using the toggle. You usually have both hands on the steering mechanism so if you pull back on the right to go forward, the left side of the toggle goes to the forward position. If your left hand is in a position such that it stops the toggle from returning to the neutral position when your right hand is no longer pulling it back, the scooter keeps going forward when you expected it to stop. This can be dangerous, e.g., when there is a dropoff in front of you. You would be surprised how easily unintended movement can happen; it happened to me several times. I was so concerned about this when I exited a Paratransit bus, where I was well above ground level, I removed my left hand from the steering mechanism completely to eliminate this risk. There are some advantages to being able to use only one side for both front and backward motion. For example, someone can control the scooter when you aren't in it without sitting on the seat by standing beside it and using only one side of the toggle to go either direction.

Considering the difficulty I had of getting up from the scooter, the risk I took at times by getting up to reach things, and my desire to learn to drive with hand controls, I realized that it was time to acquire a motorized wheelchair. The next chapter discusses how I decided what I needed, how I got insurance coverage and other important considerations.

Opposite top: **Scooter toggle at scooter rest position.** *Opposite bottom:* **Scooter toggle at forward movement position (photographs by the author).**

9

Acquiring a Wheelchair

"You need persistence in order to maintain the reality you desire."
—Steven Redhead, *Life Is a Cocktail: Reality with a Dash*
of Imagination, Shaken but Not Stirred, Please

I was not anxious to give up the scooter's advantages, but eventually, it became very difficult to get up from it. I knew it was only a matter of time before it would be impossible. Already there were times when someone had to help me get up.* There was no guarantee that there would always be someone there to assist. The intense effort to get up worried me as well. I was afraid that I would injure my legs. I was also anxious to take advantage of the capabilities that a wheelchair would provide, specifically, safer and easier transfers, the ability to reach things at elevated levels, increased travel distance, and comfort. For these reasons, I decided to acquire a wheelchair.

About that time, Joel, a member of my golf group, told me that one of the guys he target shot with used a wheelchair and was still driving. I called and started a beneficial phone and email conversation. He explained his views on the front, mid, and rear-wheel drive wheelchairs' pros and cons and mentioned some of the brands that I should consider. He also indicated that he had bought used wheelchairs online at times to reduce cost. One of the most important things he did for me was to recommend that I go to a mobility expo. Fortunately, one was coming soon nearby. It has since occurred to me that what he did for me is what I intend this book to do for others.

At that point, I couldn't drive to the expo, but Steve Steen, my continually helpful next-door neighbor, offered to be my driver. Attending the expo was extremely valuable because of what I learned and the contacts I made, which led to other contacts. I highly recommend you consider attending an expo when there is one in your area. There I test drove different wheelchairs and gathered information about them through brochures and by talking to the salespeople. One salesman worked for Access Medical, a company that represents Permobil, one of the top wheelchair manufacturers. I also spoke to a company called Mobility-Works, a company that adapts vans for disabled people who want to drive.

---

* People grab your arms to get you up but that raises your center of gravity and doesn't allow you to help with whatever leg strength you have. Have them pull up on the back of your belt instead.

The representative for MobilityWorks also provided valuable information about what type of wheelchair would work best if I planned to drive with hand controls, which was an objective I was pursuing. He recommended a mid-wheel drive wheelchair for that purpose because of its turning radius and the fact that the center of the turning circle is the center of the chair.

The next step was to see my doctor. He sent me to an occupational therapist (OT) who was also a Certified Driver Rehabilitation Specialist (CDRS®). More information on CDRS® capabilities is discussed later in this book in connection with handicapped driving. The occupational therapist evaluated me and set up a second meeting with him and a representative from Access Medical, who turned out to be the person I had met at the mobility expo. We discussed all the necessary features and the functions I thought were required, including tilt, recline, and elevation. I realized that eventually, I would probably use the wheelchair all day so I would need a good seat cushion and power leg elevation. At that meeting, I was able to test a chair with all the functions that seemed necessary.

Based on my needs and information I had gathered, I decided on a mid-wheel drive wheelchair and chose the Permobil M3 shown below.

Until I decided to obtain the wheelchair, it had not been excessively time-consuming or challenging to acquire the equipment I wanted. However, getting insurance coverage for the wheelchair was different. In the end, I was able to get the Permobil M3 and most of the controls I wanted paid for by Medicare using the process presented at the beginning of Section Three.

There are many factors to consider when acquiring a wheelchair. This chapter

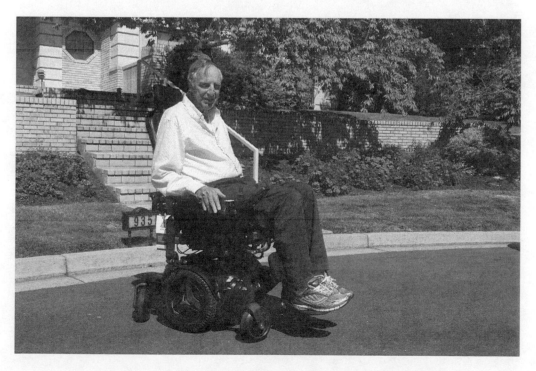

On my Permobil M3 wheelchair (photograph by Taylor Bland).

covers the many wheelchair options, their pros and cons, and the reasons for my decisions. The next chapter provides the consequences of those decisions.

Understanding the pros and cons of the options available, the obstacles I encountered, and how they were overcome should help you accomplish your goals. Listed below are the topics discussed in this chapter:

1. Wheelchair types
2. Control options
3. Getting insurance approval

Wheelchair Types

There is an incredible variety of wheelchair options, so many that you might want to get help from a specialist to make your choice. A good source for an overview of the possibilities is the United Spinal Association.[1] There are powered and manual all-terrain wheelchairs; rigid and folding manual wheelchairs; compact and full-sized powered wheelchairs; pediatric wheelchairs; positioning wheelchairs; sports wheelchairs; standing wheelchairs; and beach wheelchairs. In each of these categories, there are variations in weight, materials, etc. Most people with progressive diseases are seeking a good mobility device. Manual and powered wheelchairs are the only wheelchair options I cover in this book.

If you have good upper body strength, you will be able to use a manual wheelchair. There are many different versions. Some are heavy; others weigh only about 25 pounds. A folding chair can be put in a car; some models even fit in airplane overhead bins. Some newer versions come with a suspension system at the cost of extra weight.

I knew I had no possibility of having acceptable mobility with a manual wheelchair. I quickly settled on a motorized wheelchair. There are many versions of motorized wheelchairs, many manufacturers, and many control options that can help make your life safer and more comfortable. Some leading manufacturers of motorized wheelchairs are Pride Mobility, Permobil, and Invacare Corporation. I decided that I needed a full-size chair due to my size and the control options I needed.

A motorized wheelchair has two drive wheels. There are three- and four-wheel types. The location of the drive wheels creates three types of wheelchairs: rear-wheel, mid-wheel, and front-wheel drive. Each has advantages and disadvantages. Mobility Management[2] and the Muscular Dystrophy Association[3] are excellent resources for information on each type's advantages and disadvantages. Below is a brief overview of the different drive types.

Front-wheel drive wheelchairs are optimal when driving on unpaved areas and over small obstacles but they travel at lower speeds. The reason for this is that they are less stable and can fishtail at high speeds. Another difficulty is because most of the chair is behind you, there is more of a tendency to bump into things while maneuvering. The rear of the front-wheel-drive swings around behind you where you can't see it easily.

Rear-wheel drive wheelchairs aren't as good going over obstacles as front-wheel but can travel faster than the other options and are very stable. They have the largest turning radius. Also, because most of the chair is in front of you, you are less likely to bump into objects. They can tip back on steep slopes but have anti-tipping mechanisms to deal with that issue.

Mid-wheel drive wheelchairs are the optimum choice for use in your home as they have the tightest turning radius which is best when maneuvering in small spaces. For the same reason, mid-wheel is the best choice for transporting yourself in a van either as a passenger or a driver.

The best way to secure a chair is with an EZ Lock[4] or similar docking device. This means installing a pin under the chair which can interfere with uneven surfaces for everyday use. Because the mid-wheel versions place the pin between the drive wheels, this issue is minimized. For example, when going over a threshold the drive wheels go over a threshold at the same time as the pin so the pin goes up with the wheels. This isn't the case with front and rear-wheel drive wheelchairs.

However, mid-wheel wheelchairs are the worst choice if your primary use is outdoors, particularly if you frequently go over rough terrains, soft ground (e.g., sand) or steep slope transitions. On steep slope transitions, the drive wheels can lose contact with the ground. In such cases, the wheelchair is supported solely by the front and rear casters so the drive wheels can't move the chair. This problem can also occur in soft terrain and is unique to the mid-wheel wheelchair. They also produce the roughest ride.

I chose a mid-wheel drive wheelchair because the great majority of my usage was going to be in the home and because I planned to drive with hand controls. Maneuvering in the van would be easier with the mid-wheel version. I would be secured by an EZ Lock and would have less concern about the pin for regular use. I understood the drawbacks of this choice but I thought they were minor issues for my situation and needs. Your needs may lead you to a different choice.

Control Options

A joystick controls most wheelchairs, but there are many other ways to control the chair available to accommodate various disabilities. You can control a wheelchair with your head, chin, tongue, speech, finger, touchpad, breath, and other ways. MobilityBasics[5] describes these control options. For insurance coverage, you must show you have a medical necessity for a special control system.

This section focuses on a joystick as part of a control panel. That is what I needed and probably what most readers would want. There are many joystick and control panel variations. I chose the control panel that had separate buttons to control the wheelchair options, e.g., tilt and recline. These functions could be controlled using only the control panel and joystick, but the dedicated buttons are much easier to use. In one case I will describe later, using those buttons was important to me achieving my objective.

I chose and recommend a control panel that can be rotated outside and inside the arm on which it is mounted. This is of utmost importance as the wheelchair will have to pass through narrow areas and if you damage the control panel, the chair won't function. The repair cost can be high and damage to the chair is not covered by your health care insurance. For that reason, I recommend keeping the control panel inside the armrest most of the time to avoid damage to it, as long as it doesn't make maneuvering the chair difficult. The exception to having the controller inside or in the normal position is when you are transferring to or from the wheelchair. One will naturally reach for the wheelchair arms during transitions and, if by mistake, you push down on the control panel, it can be damaged. This is particularly true when you are transferring to the wheelchair because your back will be turned to the arms and controller when you are sitting down. Moving the control panel outside the arm during transfers will minimize that risk. See the following pictures of the control panel in the normal, inside, and outside positions.

Power wheelchairs offer many valuable control options including power tilt, power recline, power leg rest elevation, power chair elevation, and seat design. Invacare[6] has a good website for describing the value of these control options. Many other websites also provide helpful information.

In many cases, you may need to use more than one control option to accomplish your goal. Because there are both positives and negatives associated with these options, it is important to talk with an occupational therapist to determine what is best for your condition and needs. An overview of each option is presented below.

Power Tilt

Tilt rotates the chair backward and forwards, changing the seat angle relative to the ground. However, the seat to backrest angle is unchanged, as well as

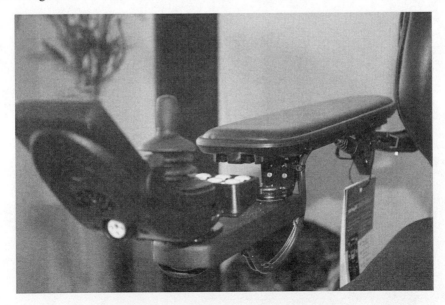

Wheelchair controller normal position (photograph by the author).

the seat to leg rest angle. Spending long hours in wheelchairs and lift chairs creates the risk of developing pressure sores, which can lead to other serious health issues. Some backward tilt helps relieve pressure and reduces the risk of pressure sores. Backward tilt also improves safety when driving downgrade or over rough surfaces. The combination of backward tilt and elevation can make it safer to use a lift to go up one or two steps because the leg rests and your feet can be placed above the step before you take the lift up. That eliminates the risk of damaging your feet or the leg rests as you are raised.

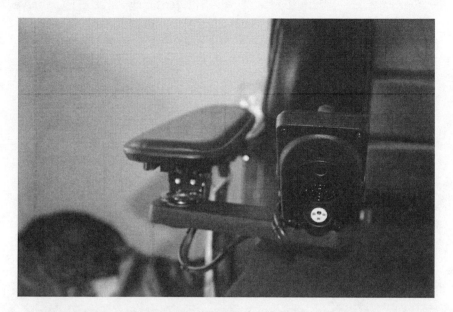

Wheelchair controller inside position (photograph by the author).

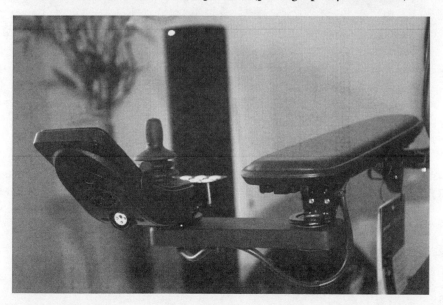

Wheelchair controller outside position (photograph by the author).

Tilting the chair down offers two valuable capabilities. The first relates to transfers. I found that a full-tilt forward, followed by an elevation up until only your toes touch the ground leads to a very easy transfer. Initially, only the toes touch, but when you slide forward on the seat the entire bottoms of your feet are on the ground. Then there isn't much effort getting to a standing position. The second capability is that it will assist you when needing to pick up items on lower surfaces.

My chair came with significant back tilt and some forward tilt. I was offered a larger forward tilt but concluded that it was unnecessary and too expensive. Note that when you change the tilt direction, the tilt angle will change until you are back to neutral and then stop. You must stop pushing the button briefly and push again to complete the tilt change desired.

Power Recline

Recline changes the backrest angle relative to the ground while maintaining a constant seat angle to the ground. The recline feature helps you find the most comfortable sitting position when sitting in the wheelchair for extended periods. A backward recline can also reduce pressure on the bottom of your body providing whole-body contact with more of the chair, thus decreasing pressure sore risk.

Reclining flat to the floor can assist with transfers to a bed. However, there are potential negative consequences to reclining back at extreme angles. For example, the body will slide forward out of position relative to the seat. It is important to consult with an occupational therapist to ensure that you get the right options for your condition and needs.

Recline is also helpful when transferring to a lift chair. The safest way to transfer to a lift chair is to move the wheelchair directly in front of the lift chair. Unfortunately, the wheelchair will then block your view of objects in front of you, such as the television, after you have transferred to the lift chair. Your view can be restored by first lowering the wheelchair to the lowest level, then tilting the chair to the neutral (flat seat) position, and then reclining nearly flat to the floor. You can also use tilt for this or in combination with recline, but it is preferable to keep the seat flat. This allows you to use the wheelchair seat for holding items while you are in the lift chair. It takes practice to unblock the view of the TV as described above because the view of the control panel is partially blocked and moved away from you. You have to establish control by feeling for the appropriate buttons. This is another good reason for having buttons to control the various motorized options. You will also need to have enough room to lay the wheelchair nearly flat in front of you for this approach to work.

The biggest drawback to this method of unblocking the TV is that it is not ideal for making a rapid return to the wheelchair. Without giving up too much safety during the transfer, I found that I could bring the wheelchair in at an angle such that it would not block the TV. This allowed me to get up from the lift chair and transfer back to the wheelchair more rapidly.

Leg Rest Elevation

The appropriate leg rest can help avoid back pain and pressure in the buttocks. The rest should have calf pads to support the legs when they are elevated. Chairs equipped with recline should also be equipped with elevating leg rests to ensure comfort. The powered leg rest is essential to safely transfer to and from the chair and for when you want to get close to something. In both cases, you need to get the leg rest out of the way. Powered leg rests are very important when you go down ramps and steep slopes because you can raise them to avoid scraping the ground. If you drive the wheelchair into the backseat of a van, you will want to raise the leg rest up to enter the van, then lower them as you turn to face forward to avoid having your feet hit the front seat. They need to be raised again to go down the ramp to exit the van.

Seat Design

Most wheelchair users spend many hours a day in their wheelchairs. A well-cushioned seat and the ability to shift your weight are needed to avoid pressure sores. Even before I got the wheelchair, my doctor was sufficiently worried about pressure sores that he ordered a salve for me. He was concerned about the time I spent in the scooter and on the lift chair.

The tilt and recline features help with weight shifting, but you still need a well-cushioned seat. There are different options to accomplish this. There are foam cushions, air cushions, gel-filled cushions, and polyurethane honeycomb cushions. More information can be found by searching on the internet for seat cushioning options for power wheelchairs. A site with good information on seat options is Hoveround.[7]

My wheelchair has an air-cushioned seat and includes a pump to change the firmness when desired. After using the wheelchair for a few months, I found a drawback to this type of seat. They tend to leak and need to be pumped up frequently. I replaced it under warranty but the replacement leaked as well. Permobil then replaced it with an air-cushioned seat that did not have a foam border like the other seats. It has worked well.

Elevation

The most important advantage of powered elevation is the ability to elevate and lower the seat to facilitate transfers to and from the wheelchair to other places, e.g., your bed, lift chair, shower chair and commode. I'd be lost without it. I can't over-emphasize its importance. I strongly recommend you buy a chair with the powered elevation. It is the most important feature.

Powered elevation makes it possible to reach things you would not have access to otherwise. For example, I gained access to the freezer, dish cabinets, etc., that had long been out of reach. This reduced my dependence on Jodie. Elevation can be used for other purposes as well. As explained in the tilt paragraph above, I use it on the lifts to avoid catching my feet or the leg rests under the lip on the higher level when going up. The elevation option is expensive and usually not covered by insurance. I know of one person who got it covered by private insurance but Medicare doesn't cover it.

I decided to purchase the wheelchair with all the options indicated earlier. I felt it was much safer for me and because being independent was a very important goal of mine.

Getting Insurance Coverage

I was warned that Medicare would not pay for elevation. We made a great effort to demonstrate that I required elevation but they still would not pay for it. You can appeal and try to get their decision overturned. Because the odds of success were very low and trying would delay the time it took to get the wheelchair, I declined to appeal.

The process of getting the paperwork to Medicare became extremely time consuming and frustrating. As mentioned earlier, when I got Medicare approval for my rolling walker, I had my neurologist work with a physical therapist to file the paperwork that would work. I also had several conversations with the supplier before I got the exact walker I wanted.

I then learned a long and trying lesson of the importance of maintaining a relationship with the neurologist who first diagnosed your condition. My not doing this caused much time delay and frustration when working with Medicare. As your situation evolves, you will need different equipment and other types of help. The best way to ensure you receive this is by establishing a continuing relationship with your neurologist. I highly recommend this.

My neurologist had helped get approval for the rolling walker and for the use of the Paratransit system, which is discussed later in the book. I had already seen an occupational therapist, so my next step was to get an appointment with my neurologist. She could sign the paperwork so we could file for Medicare approval. However, when I went to make an appointment, I was told that, since I hadn't seen her for quite a while, I was going to be treated as a new patient. Normally that would delay things many months, but it was worse than that. She wasn't accepting new patients.

It was true that I hadn't seen her for some time. She had told me that I had two untreatable diseases and there was nothing they could do for me. I didn't see the point of having more appointments but that turned out to be a mistake. I should have realized that I would continue to evolve and need different equipment and other types of help as my situation changed.

Since I didn't have a neurologist to sign off on Medicare's paperwork, I elected to use my general practitioner (GP). I was a little concerned about that because he had referred me to a neurologist when I asked for his help getting the walker. However, he understood that I no longer had a neurologist but knew that I urgently needed a wheelchair and agreed to help. It took a lot longer than I anticipated to coordinate with the OT and Access Medical to finalize the paperwork and get an appointment with my GP.

The paperwork sent to the doctor from the OT and Access Medical included a suggested Medicare code. The doctor read through all the paperwork and was more than willing to sign the documents, but he thought the code wasn't quite right. He crossed it out, put in two new codes, and initialed the changes, explaining that although all the codes should work, the codes he substituted were more precise.

I was elated that we finally got this done and called my contact at Access Medical with the great news. There was a long pause before he said: "He changed the code?" I repeated that he had and gave him the codes the doctor used. He looked them up and said, to my surprise: "That's not going to work. You won't get Medicare to approve this." He then sent me a document that listed all the codes Medicare would have accepted. My first thought was: "Why didn't he send this to me before I went to see the doctor?" Within minutes of learning this, I tried to contact the doctor as he seemed to feel that the original code would probably work, but the only response I got was a referral to another neurologist. Once he had put a different code on the paperwork, he was reluctant to do anything else. I understood that but now faced another potentially long delay.

When I called the neurologist he recommended, I found that it would be a long time before I could see him and was getting very concerned about my ability to get up from the scooter much longer. I called my original neurologist's office again to see if they would make an exception. They wouldn't but offered another neurologist who wasn't as heavily booked. I had to wait to see her too but she was extremely cooperative. I showed her the list of codes that would work after explaining what had happened with my GP. She agreed with my doctor that the original code was not correct but looked through the codes I provided and found two consistent with my medical condition. She said that she would sign the papers if we sent her the paperwork with the corrected codes. Despite a little trouble coordinating the OT and Access Medical, the necessary document was received and signed by the neurologist.

Even this overly long description does not fully convey the length of time and frustration associated with getting effective paperwork sent to Medicare. I provided this level of detail to reinforce that you need both patience and persistence to get through this. You must continue to be your own advocate. If you have a neurologist and know what insurance codes will work before your appointment, it will avoid much of the delay I experienced.

Even after all of the work preparing the application, Medicare didn't approve it in the normal time requirement. Instead, they sent questions that had to be answered. Then they approved everything except the elevation option, which was expected. Using Medicare saved about $20,000 vs. purchasing it on my own. The effort and frustration were worth it but could have been avoided if I had maintained a relationship with my neurologist and been provided a list of codes before I saw my GP or the neurologist.

My aim with this book is to help you avoid these roadblocks, so I have included a list of codes that I believe will work if you are on Medicare. Your neurologist or doctor may have enough knowledge and experience that they won't need it. The salesperson who is selling you the chair might also have a list. In any case, you should have the list. You can show it to your neurologist or ask what code they think applies and check it against the list. The list is presented below.

As has been demonstrated in this book, getting insurance coverage for medical equipment can be very challenging. However, I have been successful

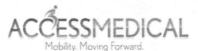

COMMON NEUROLOGIC CONDITIONS	ICD-10	HEMIPLEGIA/HEMIPARESIS (cont.)	ICD-10
Alzheimer's Disease	G30.9	(Post-Polio) Late Effect Acute Polio	G14
Other Inherited Spinal Muscular Atrophy	G12.1	Concentric Sclerosis (Balo) of Central Nervous System	G37.5
Amyotrophic Lateral Sclerosis	G12.21	Diffuse Sclerosis of Central Nervous System	G37.0
Central Demyelination of Corpus Callosum	G37.1	Schilder's Disease	G37.0, G37
Central Pontine Myelinolysis	G37.2	SPINAL CORD INJURY	
CEREBRAL PALSY		Quadriplegia, Unspecific	G82.50
Spastic Diplegic Cerebral Palsy	G80.1	Quadriplegia, C1-C4 Complete	G82.51
Spastic Hemiplegic Cerebral Palsy	G80.2	Quadriplegia, C1–C4 Incomplete	G82.52
Spastic Quadriplegic Cerebral Palsy	G80.0	Quadriplegia, C5-C7 Complete	G82.53
Other Cerebral Palsy	G80.8	Quadriplegia, C5-C7 Incomplete	G82.54
Cerebral Palsy, Unspecified	G80.9	Paraplegia, NOS	G82.20
Early –Onset Cerebral Ataxia	G11.1	Diplegia of Upper Extremity	G83.0
Tay-Sachs Disease	E75.02	Spinocerebellar Disease	G11.9
Neuronal Ceroidlipofuscinosis	E75.4	Spinal Muscular Atrophy	G12.9
Congenital Nonprogressive Ataxia	G11.0	Symptomatic Torsion Dystonia	G24.2
Late-Onset Cerebral Ataxia	G11.2	Spinocerebellar Disease NEC G11.9, G11.13, G11.8	
Encepalitis, Myelitis, and Encephalomyelitis	G05	Syringomyelia	G95.0
Guillian Barre	G61.0	Traumatic Brain Injury – Quadriplegia	G82.50
HEMIPLEGIA/HEMIPARESIS		Vascular Myelopathies	G95.19
Flaccid Hemiplegia Affecting Unspecified Side	G81.00	Werdnig-Hoffman's Disease	G12.0
Flaccid Hemiplegia and Hemiparesis RIGHT G81.01, LEFT G81.02 Affecting Dominant Side			
Flaccid Hemiplegia Affecting Non - Dominant Side	RIGHT G81.03, LEFT G81.04	MYOPATHY	
		Congenital Myopathy	G71.2
Spastic Hemiplegia Unspecified Side	G81.10	Dermatomyositis (Wagners)	M33.90
Spastic Hemiplegia Dominant Side	RIGHT G81.11, LEFT G81.12	Myasthenia Gravis	G70.00
Spastic Hemiplegia Non- Dominant Side	RIGHT G81.13, LEFT G81.14	Myotonia Congenital	G71.12
		Myositis Ossificans	M61.10
Spastic Hemiplegia Cerebral Palsy	G80.2	MUSCULAR DYSTROPHY	
Hereditary Spastic Paraplegia	G11.4	Beckers	G71.0
Huntington's Chorea	G10	Duchennes	G71.0
Idiopathic Torsion Dystonia	G24.1	Polymyositis	M33.20
Kugelberg-Welander Disease	G12.1	Polymyositis Ossificans	M61.59
Metachromatic Leukodystrophy	E75.25	Myositis, Unspecified M60.9, M79.1, M79.	
Myelopathy in Other Disease	G99.2		
Motor Neuron NEC	G12.29	CONGENITAL SKELETAL DEFORMITY	
Multiple Sclerosis	G35	Congenital Dislocation of Unspecified	Q65.00
Parkinson's Disease	G20	Klinefelters Syndrome Q98.4 Osteogenesis Imperfec	
Amyotrophic Lateral Sclerosis	G12.21	Q78.0	
Pseudo Bulbar Palsy	G12.22	Spinal Bifida with Hydrocephalus	Q05.4
Primary lateral Sclerosis	G12.29	Spina Bifida	Q05

Medicare codes (provided by Access Medical).

using the procedure provided in the introduction to Section Three. It should help you.

When it wasn't clear that I would receive insurance coverage, I searched and found a used version of the same model of the wheelchair I wanted online. It was manufactured a year earlier but hadn't been used very much. It had a lot of features that I wanted but not all of the important ones. I learned that it is expensive to add features to a wheelchair after it is built. A used chair also raised a question about how difficult it would be to get it serviced. Nevertheless, it is possible to save money by buying a used model.

The next chapter discusses the consequences of wheelchair use.

10

The Consequences
of Wheelchair Use

"You may encounter many defeats, but you must not be defeated. In fact, it may be necessary to encounter the defeats, so you can know who you are, what you can rise from, how you can still come out of it."
—Maya Angelou

Using a wheelchair for mobility is not free of issues. Each of the considerations listed below are discussed in this chapter.

1. Access
2. Safety
3. Transporting Items
4. Getting Close
5. Capital Cost
6. Maintenance Cost
7. Convenience

Access

We decided to stay in our home and have the doors widened to allow the wheelchair to access the rooms. We love our home, the views, our neighbors and friends, and the location. The house had already been modified in some ways to accommodate my limitations, such as installing lifts, building a special shower room, installing grab bars, etc. We would also incur a substantial capital gain if we sold the house, which could be avoided or minimized if one or both of us died while we still owned the home.

Safety

There are three primary safety concerns. The first is potential foot injury because the feet are unprotected in a wheelchair. You will inevitably hit your feet. Always wear shoes, which will limit the damage, and be vigilant. Go slowly and watch your feet. Your upper leg can hide them. You will need to move your head until you can see your feet as you get close to possible obstacles. Also, when maneuvering near obstacles, lower your speed setting because the chair won't stop suddenly. At slower speeds, it will stop sooner. There is no brake; stopping depends on the motor's inertia. The faster you go, the greater the stopping distance. Even after I had used the wheelchair for many months, I occasionally misjudged this and hurt my feet. You also need to be cautious while turning the chair. I have hit my feet numerous times while turning.

The second safety concern is avoiding unintended movement. It is best to turn off the wheelchair during transfers and anytime you are stopped, particularly if you plan to reach for something. It is very easy to move the joystick and get sudden, unexpected movement. Also, your clothing can catch on the joystick and move the wheelchair dangerously. This happened to me several times in the first week. I know of one case where clothing caught on the joystick caused the wheelchair to drop off an edge, causing two broken legs. If you are close to something when the joystick moves, you could damage your chair or yourself. It is best to avoid reaching for objects when the chair is powered. However, sometimes you can just move the controller away from the direction you intend to reach without turning it off if you do it carefully.

The third safety concern relates to the problem with casters when changing direction. Because they need to be oriented to face the direction the chair is moving, the casters spin. When you change from forward movement to backward movement or vice versa, the casters point other ways than intended until completing their spin. During this process, the wheelchair will move in unintended ways. In tight spaces, this can cause impacts. I learned the hard way to avoid or minimize this problem by always starting very slowly when changing direction. If you are in a tight or dangerous place, "feather" the movement. By feathering, I mean move and release the joystick quickly many times until the casters have completed the spin. This way you won't be pushed too far in the wrong direction as the casters turn.

In my first week, while exiting the kitchen door to get on the garage lift, the slightly raised threshold caused the front casters to take a hard right and the chair spun. I was stuck! The right wheels were up hard against a 2×4 stop on the right to avoid a drop-off. On the left side, the chair was hard up against the doorway. The chair wouldn't move either way. I got out of this by repeatedly kicking the casters in different directions, then moving a little each time.

Even after I had been using my wheelchair for a month and had better control of it, I had a more serious problem with the caster movement. I had gone into a tight space between the kitchen table and the kitchen counter and then had to reverse direction. The caster movement caused the wheelchair to lurch hard into the kitchen counter, trapping my arm between the chair and the counter. A large patch of skin was torn off of my arm. I had forgotten to use the feathering method to get the casters realigned for the backward movement.

Transporting Items

I was able to find a solution for carrying things like my wallet, keys, eyeglasses, sunglasses, garage door opener, etc. Permobil sells an underarm organizer that does not increase the width of the chair. It costs about $150 which I thought was excessive. I found a Sammons Preston Under Arm Organizer on Amazon for $33 that works as well or better. All my essential items fit nicely into the front slip-in compartment or the larger compartment. It was fully satisfactory for my needs. The larger pocket has two zippers, so one can zip both sides up and leave the top open, making it easy to put things in or take them out. The only drawback is because of my wheelchair's wide arms, the only way I could install the organizer was to put it together and slide it on the arm from the front. That meant that I could not put it on the arm that had the controller.

The front and side views of the organizer appear below.

In cold weather, the scooter can carry extra garments in the front basket. This was very useful in case Jodie got cold or the wind intensified. I found no acceptable answer to that with the wheelchair except to hold the extra garments in my lap.

Getting Close

With a scooter, I got close to tables by either coming in at the end of the table or by removing one chair from a round table or two chairs from the side of

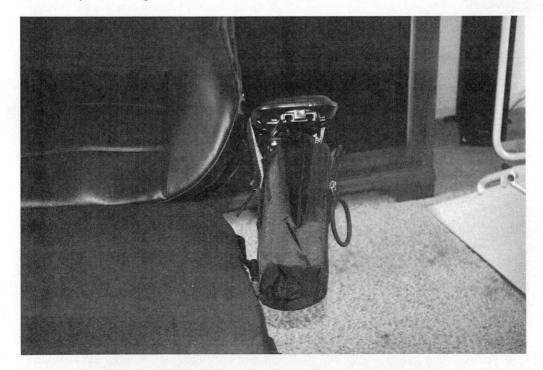

Wheelchair organizer front view (photograph by the author).

a rectangular table and turning the seat 90 degrees. That won't work for a wheelchair. You will need access to the table and be able to pull under it slightly. You need about 30 inches between the table's legs and 30 inches from the floor to the table's underside. Also, the aisle needs to be about 36 inches wide.

It's best to call and ask questions if you are going to an unfamiliar restaurant. I found most restaurants are designed to accommodate wheelchairs fitting under the table. Among the websites providing information on this are Tablebases.com[1] and Karman Healthcare, Inc.[2] You might want to modify some counters in your home so you can drive the wheelchair under them.

Capital Cost

If you have a medical reason to need a wheelchair and follow the procedure presented earlier, most or all of the cost will be covered unless you choose the elevation option.

Maintenance Cost

According to Access Medical who sold me the chair, the first service needed should be in approximately one and a half years and would be for tires and general maintenance items. The warranty is for one year. The controller and motors

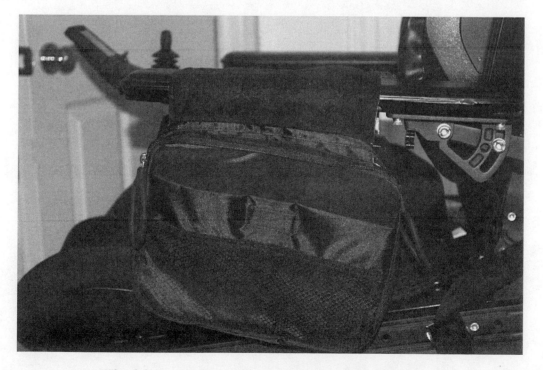

Wheelchair organizer side view (photograph by the author).

are usually good for four to five years. However, this is an electrically-powered device with many controls; things can go wrong. Maintenance costs are covered by your health insurance after one year, in my case Medicare. My wheelchair has gel-cell lead-acid batteries which are designed to be maintenance-free and there is no chance of chemical spilling. Karman Healthcare, Inc.[3] provides some maintenance cost estimates for motors, joysticks, and other items.

Convenience

With gel-cell batteries, wheelchairs can go on planes. Southwest Airlines told me they take it up a ramp through a wide door. They have to recline the chair due to the height but that is not a problem. The challenge is to be able to transport the chair at the other end of your flight. A first step would be to check to see if there is something like Paratransit that can take you to your destination. With enough notice, an accessible van can be rented from MobilityWorks, United Access or similar firms at your destination. It is unlikely they will have the controls you need to enable you to drive if you are a disabled driver but a relative, friend or business associate could pick up the van, meet you at the airport, and take you to your destination. When you are ready to go home, that person can take you back to the airport and return the van.

Here are a few other useful facts about wheelchairs.

1. There are switches on my wheelchair that can disconnect the motor from the wheels so that the wheelchair can be pushed. I had a similar capability on my scooter but the scooter weighed substantially less, making this a desirable option. The more extended range of the wheelchair makes this potential need much less critical but it could be useful in rare cases. However, pushing an occupied motorized wheelchair that might weigh 600 lbs is challenging, especially uphill.

2. There are four obvious receptors for locking devices on the wheelchair for use when traveling on Paratransit or in my van's back seat. My scooter didn't have these and was secured in various ways, some of which concerned me.

3. If you fully elevate the chair, the speed of travel will automatically be reduced by half for safety. Fully elevating the chair and maximizing tilt will stop the wheelchair from moving at all for safety reasons.

4. My wheelchair can connect through Bluetooth to Permobil's app so they can track any problems with the equipment. Privacy issues could be a concern, but in case of an emergency, I want to be able to call and get a diagnosis at once. I had a problem with my scooter twice when I was away from home, and as it did not have that option, it was difficult to get answers.

5. My wheelchair has a switch that will disconnect the battery from the electrical system which might be useful if you weren't going to use it for a long time, but it isn't well designed for disabled people. I can turn it off, but not on, so it is useless to me.

6. I now had some access to the cabinets in the kitchen, but not the ability to take heavy things down from the second or third level. Also, without the ability to reach far enough back into the shelves on the first level for some items, that capability was more limited than I expected. I could have paid for more forward tilt but I felt the cost wasn't justified and it also would raise some safety issues.

7. You will find that wheelchairs and throw-rugs that lay loose aren't compatible. Throw rugs can get bunched up and caught up in the wheelchair. The casters can change directions when going over a bunched rug and take you in a direction different than you intended. It is best to remove these rugs to eliminate the above possibilities, and I did so from our kitchen.

8. There are also problems with wheelchairs and carpets, though not as severe. Because of the weight of a wheelchair and the ability to make tight turns, the carpets will stretch, move and possibly ripple. If possible, avoid tight turns and move slightly in one direction or another as you turn. It is also more difficult moving on a carpet, which sometimes will require an increase in speed to move.

9. You only have to charge the wheelchair battery once a day, at night, and then only if you have used it extensively. My wheelchair is placed near my bed nightly when I transfer from it to the walker and then into the bed. While it is beside the bed, I can charge the battery when needed.

There is one more chapter in this section on personal mobility. The previous chapters have identified and evaluated the various devices, e.g., canes, walkers, scooters, and wheelchairs that can help achieve mobility. However, having level changes in the home can make those devices ineffective. The final chapter of this section describes the solutions available to achieve personal mobility if your home has level changes and these solutions' implications.

11

Dealing with
House Level Changes

"The greater the obstacle, the more glory in overcoming it."
—Molière

This chapter discusses how to deal with two different types of home level changes. Multi-story homes have multiple steps to higher living space levels. Another type has level changes that involve a step up or down to some parts of the home. Frequently, these are referred to as single-level homes, but they are not. A single-level home means that all areas of the home are on the same level.

If your home has more than one level and you currently have mobility challenges or a diagnosis that indicates that they are in your future, it is best to move to a one-level home before you start incurring significant costs to accommodate your needs. However, there are often compelling reasons to stay in your home as long as you can. Living close to family and friends could be one of them. Your house, grounds, and location might make you reluctant to leave. If you are a caregiver for a family member, moving to a strange location could devastate them, an important consideration. Your ability to incur significant renovation costs without creating a financial hardship must also be considered.

The decision to move could be one of the most difficult you ever have to make. As soon as you get a diagnosis, talk to the neurologist about what you can expect and when. Then decide which course of action is best and proceed to act on it.

If your home has multiple stories and your mobility device is a walker, scooter or wheelchair, the only practical way to live there is to never go to the second story. There are stairlifts but if you use a mobility device or likely soon will, you won't be able to move safely on the second level without a second mobility device to use there. Also, you have to be able to get up from the chair of a stairlift. You may not be able to get up without assistance, particularly long-term.

Another important consideration, depending on your staircase, a stairlift can cost $3,000 to $10,000. Medicare typically won't cover the cost because they consider them a home modification, not covered by their guidelines. If you decide to install a stairlift, check with your insurance provider to see whether it is covered. Medicaid might cover it in your state.

101mobility.com[1] has information on funding sources that could be of interest. You can find more information on stairlifts by searching on the Internet. Most people with progressive disease will be unlikely to want a stairlift because it would be a short-term solution with significant disadvantages. Accordingly, this chapter is focused on one or two-step level changes rather than multi-story homes.

In a one or two-level change home, the limited number of level changes make living there more feasible. Even so, you have to be very motivated to remain in your home and then be able to deal with the costs and negatives of the solutions. With progressive disease, your needs may change slowly, so it is easy to make incremental changes, but the cost will add up over time. If you finally decide to move, not only will you have incurred a high cost, but the modifications made to the house will likely make the home less desirable to potential buyers.

Ramps are the best solution if it is reasonable to install them. Since they aren't mechanical and are not electrically operated, virtually nothing can go wrong; no maintenance is required. A crucial benefit is that a power outage does not render them useless, unlike electrically powered lifts. The main problem is the space they require. Even if there is room, it can be very inconvenient to have them stick out so far into the room.

The Americans with Disabilities Act (ADA) recommends a 1:12 slope, so every 1" of vertical rise requires at least 12" of ramp length. The usual step height in a home is ~7.5", so the length of the ramp would be about 7'6". If that works in your home, you will save a lot of money vs. installing a lift and will not have to worry about maintenance. Besides, you will be able to use it during power outages. This is extremely important during emergencies.

There are many manufacturers to choose from including, Prairie View Industries, Ruedamann, Titan, and Goplus. I was able to use a threshold ramp and another ramp to go out of the family room to the two-level patio behind the house. I chose a Prairie View Industries (PVI) 24" × 36" threshold wheelchair ramp which has a 600 lb weight capacity and can accommodate a maximum of 4" rise. The weight capacity was good for the scooter and okay for the wheelchair. It cost me $157 on Amazon.

For the step down to the lower level of the patio, I chose a PVI Portable Multi-fold Ramp, 8' × 30" with an 800 lb weight capacity, which was more than enough capacity for both mobility devices. It cost me $350 on Amazon. At these prices vs. the cost of a lift, you may decide to accept inconvenience if the ramp(s) fit(s). A picture of both ramps is shown in the image on the following page.

Lifts may be your only option. In my house, both the family room and the living room are sunken by one step. Unfortunately, ramps wouldn't work inside my house due to the space required for them. Space requirements also ruled out a ramp to the garage, which is down two steps. My only option was to use lifts. They are expensive but don't require much maintenance. Failure is usually due to solenoids, electromagnet control devices, which can be replaced. Lifts don't take up as much room as ramps but are still intrusive. Manufacturers include Mac's Lift Gate Inc., Porch Lift, EZ-ACCESS, and Harmar. Prices range from $4,200 to

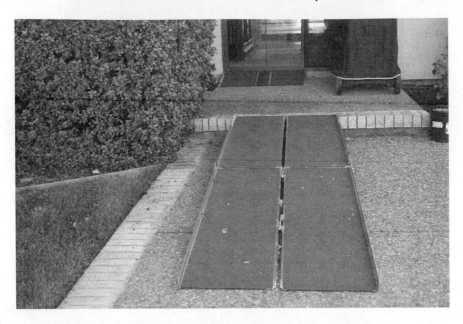

Ramps from house to patio (photograph by the author).

$6,600 per lift. I purchased three Mac's Lift Gate Inc. lifts. The pictures below show one of these lifts.

Two lifts were used in my family room to rise one step to the upper levels. One was used to get to the kitchen and dining room. The other went to the front hall, bedrooms, and bathrooms. I decided not to get one to go from the hall down

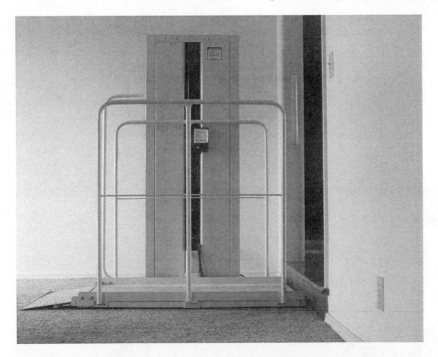

Family room lift to bedroom/bath level, side view (photograph by Anna Ericson).

to the living room. I did not use that room very often and would have had to move furniture to make it work. That saved money but there are times I regret not being able to access that room. The third lift was used to go two steps down from the kitchen to the garage.

Lifts work well but are problematic in blackouts and emergencies. They are electrically operated and there is no battery backup. There is a hand crank, but that is time-consuming and difficult to operate for a person on a mobility device. I was able to use the hand crank with the scooter on the lift, but it is a slow, tough process. I cannot use the hand crank with a wheelchair. The only other answer is a backup electrical power system.

Backup electrical power systems are discussed in the next section, focusing on issues that will help you maintain an independent life.

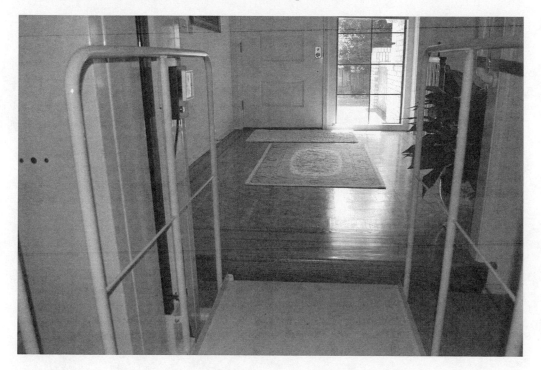

Family room lift to bedroom/bath level, front wiew (photograph by the author).

Independent Life

"You have come a long way and have won many battles.
Whenever you're faced with a difficult or challenging situation,
you'll overcome it. Yes, you can."
—Roy T. Bennett, *The Light in the Heart*

There are six chapters in this section. All of them are intended to help you maintain as much independence as possible as you encounter challenges performing normal activities in life.

1. Chapter 12 suggests ways to prepare for emergencies.
2. Chapter 13 discusses one of the most dangerous activities that you might have to perform many times a day and night, standing and transferring from one apparatus to another.
3. Chapter 14 provides a potential progression of equipment that might be necessary for toiletry.
4. Methods, equipment and home modifications that might be necessary to shower safely are all covered in Chapter 15.
5. Chapter 16 addresses the various ways to ensure that you have sufficient food and other necessities available at all times.
6. Chapter 17 suggests how to deal with various daily issues that might come up.

12

How to Prepare
for Emergencies

*"Life requires thorough preparation. Veneer isn't worth anything;
we must disabuse our people of the idea that there is a short cut to
achievement."*
—George Washington Carver, quoted in Raleigh H. Merritt,
*From Captivity to Fame: or the Life of
George Washington Carver* (1929)

Everyone should prepare for emergencies, but anticipating problems is essential and possibly life saving for people with chronic diseases. When problems occur, you need to be able to get assistance immediately. The primary advice is always to have your cell phone within reach, even when you are home. However, when you call 911, the operator has little information about you except what you provide them at that time and your general location.

There is a better solution! It is the Smart911 system,[1] which I highly recommend. Smart911 is a service many communities now support. It is an app that allows you to input critical information that you might not be able to provide when an emergency occurs. You can enter information about your medical condition, allergies, medical equipment, emergency contacts, medications, and much more. You decide what you want to provide. Once you create a profile, when you call 911, your information will then automatically display on the dispatcher's 911 screen. The dispatcher immediately has critical information that can be provided to the first responders that they might not get otherwise. It is a national service so your Smart911 profile is visible to any participating 911 center nationwide. According to Smart911, "Over 80% of calls made to 9–1–1 come from mobile phones." You are much safer if you both keep a cell phone nearby and have signed up for Smart911.

My profile has information about Jodie and me, including pictures, birthdates, address, physical descriptions, blood types, allergies, medical conditions, location of Advance Directives, emergency contacts, license plate number, description of my van, etc. It is also possible to attach PDF files. I attached medical histories for us.

While having your cell phone with you is essential and will suffice in most situations, it is highly unlikely that you will have it available at all times. Even if you do, your cell battery charge might be too low to work or you could be in an area with no cell service. For those reasons, you should also obtain a medical alert device. Such a device can help with medical emergencies and can lead to a faster response. To be safe, the medical alert device should be on your body. I recommend a mobile-based system that can work inside or outside your home. Since they have GPS, your location will be known. A monitored system is best but there are other options. Consumer Reports has an informative article, "How to Choose a Medical Alert System,"[2] on the choices and what you should consider before making a decision.

The cell phone or medical alert device is the first step to call for help but is not always sufficient. That help must be able to reach you, and if your house is locked that could be a serious problem. The solution is to acquire a Knox Box.[3] A Knox Box is a device that you install near your front door. Only your local fire department will have a key to open and lock the device. This will allow firefighters to access your home for fire or medical emergencies. The link in the footnote will enable you to see the options available and place an order.[*] As I found that the website had a flaw preventing me from accessing the cart to purchase the Knox Box, I also included the company's phone number in the footnote.

The key to open the box is fire department specific. You must be sure to call your fire department before you order. After you receive and install the box, notify the fire department. They will then insert your home key and lock the box. The picture at the top of the following page shows a fireman opening the Knox Box and the house key inside. The picture below it shows it closed.

While the lady from the fire department was locking my key in the Knox Box, I informed her that I wanted the dispatchers to know that I have both a nerve disease and a muscle disease and Jodie has dementia. Because of the Health Insurance Portability and Accountability Act of 1996 (HIPAA) privacy requirements, I had to give her written authorization to provide this information to the dispatcher. We discussed the tension between legal protection of privacy regarding medical information and the need for first responders to know what they might have to deal with in an emergency. It was after authorizing the release of our medical conditions to our local first responders that I found out about Smart911. If your community does not support Smart911 or you choose not to use Smart911, you might want to provide medical information for the first responders.

There is another option for providing vital information to first responders. This is the Vial of Life Project,[†] a Division of the Bridge Building Foundation, which has a form that you can fill out with vital information. You put the form into a baggie along with pertinent medical information and documents, e.g., a living will. The baggie and a decal provided by the foundation are then to be placed on the front of your refrigerator. A second decal is placed on your front door. This will alert the first responders that your information is available to them on the refrigerator.

---

[*] https://www.knoxbox.com/Products/Residential-KnoxBoxes/; 623-687-2300x570.

[†] For more information visit http://www.vialoflife.com.

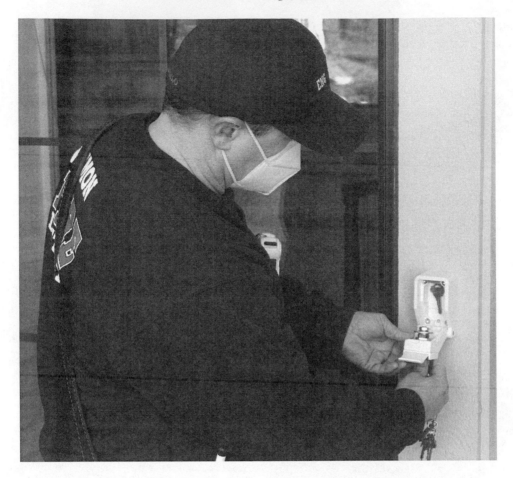

Fireman opening Knox Box, house key inside (photograph by Anna Ericson).

You can choose to have Vial of Life maintain and also store your information online as well.

If you have electrically operated lifts in your house or you are dependent on a respirator or other electrically operated equipment, it is wise to consider installing a backup electrical power system. Such a system is powered by gasoline, propane, or natural gas, so it must be located outside. It can either be a system that is started manually or one programmed to come on automatically when the power fails.

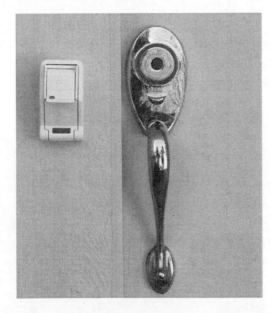

Fire department Knox Box closed (photograph by the author).

A manual start doesn't help if you need to operate a lift to get outside. Also, disabled people might have difficulty starting the system. The safest decision is having the backup power come on automatically.

Many other decisions concerning the backup system have to be made. Do you choose to power only certain rooms, such as the rooms with lifts and necessary medical equipment and the garage, or do you power the whole home? What fuel will you use for the generator? Factors that must be considered are cost, the type of emergency common to your location, the likely duration that you must plan for and whether you have natural gas as well as electricity at your home.

I had electrical power and natural gas and initially planned to have a system that would, in the case of lost electrical power, automatically switch first to natural gas and, if gas were unavailable, then to propane. We live in an earthquake prone area so we could lose both electricity and natural gas for an extended period. If the system could not automatically switch to gas and then, if needed, to propane, it would not be sufficient to have natural gas as the primary backup fuel; propane would be better.

The issues became:

- How big should the propane tank be?
- Would it be possible to get propane delivered after a major earthquake?
- How do those factors affect the decision on partial-home or whole-home backup?
- It would be necessary to power the refrigerator for food preservation in an extended outage.

Currently, California law requires all garage door openers sold and installed in the state to have a battery backup. This law was broadly supported because, during the major wildfire season of 2017, five people died because they couldn't open their garage doors. They couldn't get their cars out of the garage; without a car, they had no way to evacuate. They could not open the garage doors manually or didn't know how to disconnect the openers to open them manually. Neither of my openers had battery backup when I sought quotes for backup power. I had to wait over a month for one of the quotes. By that time, one garage door opener had to be replaced. The garage door problem solved, I would still have to have power backup to use one or more lifts to get to the garage floor. Also, we had a second refrigerator in the garage which had to be considered.

I concluded that I should only provide backup power to the room with the two lifts and the garage. I also decided that propane should be the backup fuel. There were multiple reasons for these decisions. I could not depend on natural gas being available after an earthquake. By powering only essential items, I would be able to have a smaller propane tank and wouldn't have to be concerned about running out of propane. We could evacuate if it looked like power would be out for a long time, propane was running low, and propane deliveries were not available. Also, the capital cost would be much lower. For more information on power generation options, read the "Generator Buying Guide"[4] by Consumer Reports.

In my case, plans had to be reviewed by the town and the fire department.

Consult with your town and fire department on their requirements as well as your electric utility if you plan to install a backup power supply.

Having made the decisions about backup power, I was ready to select a company to install it. But progressive diseases often disrupt the plans we make. Jodie's condition deteriorated and dictated that we move to a senior care facility. We chose one near our son's home in Arizona, which has allowed us to have a better family life and has provided the support we need. Because we hope to be able to return for part of the year, Jodie's condition allowing, we are not selling our home. If we can come back, I will have backup power installed before we return.

Taking some of the steps recommended in this chapter will help you in case of emergencies. The next chapter will help you safely stand and transfer between locations and devices.

13

Stand and Transfer Safely

*"Hoping for the best, prepared for the worst, and unsurprised by any-
thing in between."*
—Maya Angelou, *I Know Why the Caged Bird Sings*

With progressive disease, getting up from chairs, beds, toilets, etc., becomes
more difficult over time. Transferring from one place to another can be the risk-
iest thing you do. In previous chapters, I have discussed some of these situations
and methods to deal with them. This chapter will cover standing up and transferring in more detail and suggest the equipment and approaches that can be helpful.

Lift Chair

One of the first indicators of declining strength is difficulty getting up from
chairs. The first device that I bought to cope with this problem was a lift chair. I
purchased a Golden Technologies power lift and recliner chair in January 2013
for $2,067. As I didn't have a diagnosis of a muscle or nerve disease at the time of
purchase, I paid for it myself. Purchasing a lift chair is a great solution. The chair
has advantages beyond comfort and the ability to help you get up. An important
one is that its multiple positions allow you to transfer your weight, which helps
avoid pressure sores. Having a lift chair provides you with a very effective way to
transfer from the chair to any of your mobility devices. It also provides a place to
store eyeglasses, scissors, the TV remote, etc., as it has a large pocket on the right.
Pride, La-Z-Boy, Golden, Perfect Sleep Chair and others manufacture lift chairs.

Getting up and transferring from the lift chair remained relatively easy until
April 2019 when I lost more strength. I felt having a higher chair would solve that
problem and had my handyman, Tom Busta, build a 3¼" elevated platform using
2" by 6" pieces of wood sandwiched between ⅝" sheets of plywood. He installed
the lift chair on top of the platform. It was an inexpensive way to achieve more
height, costing only $150, and has worked very well. A picture of the platform is
shown on the next page.

Two motors control the chair for lifting and tilting. The chair has a battery backup. However, the control buttons I usually use run both motors simultaneously. The backup battery can't handle that load. Fortunately, other control

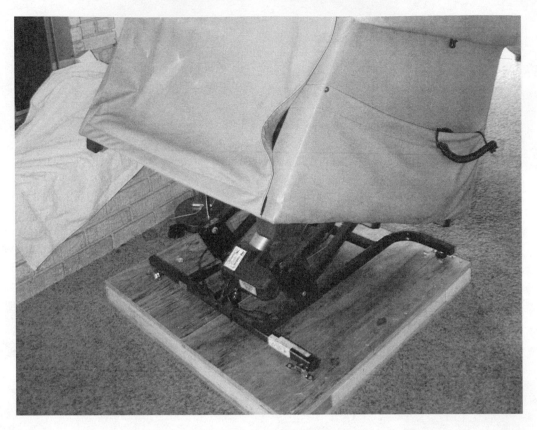

Lift chair elevated on platform (photograph by the author).

buttons use only one motor at a time. The backup batteries can lift me slowly when only one motor is applied. The first time we lost power was at night. We were in the dark, and Jodie was unable to find either a flashlight or candle. I learned two lessons from this. I now store batteries within easy reach of the chair and keep at least two flashlights beside it. Later, when the scooter was my mobility device, I simply turned on the battery-controlled scooter headlight.

If you buy the chair from a local medical equipment dealer, find out immediately who they recommend for repairs. I have had only one breakdown which occurred in late June 2016, three years and five months later. I was not able to use the chair until it was repaired. I obtained the name of a repairman from my equipment supplier. The chair was repaired quickly for $95. As the repairman would want to get additional referrals from the supplier, he was very responsive and his charge was reasonable.

Because my diseases are progressive, no solution is permanent. After I finished writing this book, I experienced another decline in strength before I sent it to publishers. Six years and three months passed before I had to put the lift chair on the 3¼" platform. But only 14 months later, in June 2020, I struggled mightily to get up from my lift chair again.

At that time, we were living in Arizona in a senior living facility; COVID-19 was peaking, and we were quarantined in our apartment. My son, Mike, and one of his friends built a platform similar to the first. The facility maintenance personnel installed it.

Transferring from the Scooter

Transferring from a walker is easy because you are already in a standing position. It is also easy to transfer from a wheelchair, particularly with elevation and tilt. Because of the scooter's lower height, it is much more difficult to transfer from the scooter to a lift chair, bed and other places. That was never easy for me and became more difficult over time. I found a technique to extend the time I was able to make this transfer. The pictures demonstrate a transfer to a lift chair and apply to all transfers from a scooter. Following the pictures, is an explanation of what each picture demonstrates in this process.

In the first photo, I have positioned my legs out in front with knees slightly bent because the objective is to straighten the legs and walk them back under me eventually. In the second photo, I am leaning forward to get the center of gravity closer to my feet as I lift with my arms.

In the third photo, my

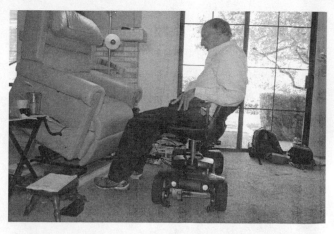

Scooter to lift chair #1, legs in front, knees bent (photograph by Taylor Bland).

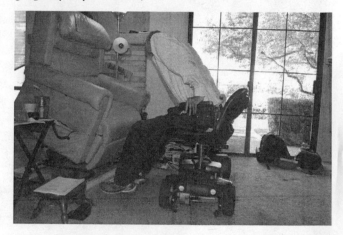

Scooter to lift chair #2, changing center of gravity (photograph by Taylor Bland).

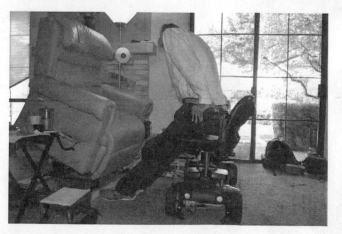

Scooter to lift chair #3, legs straight, coming up (photograph by Taylor Bland).

legs are straight and I am coming up from the scooter but have not moved my feet yet. In the fourth photo, my knees are hyper-flexed backward so I am not dependent on muscles to hold me up and I have partially walked my feet back under my shoulders.

In the fifth photo, I am off the chair with my feet walked back under my shoulders and legs hyper-flexed backward ready for transfer. In the sixth photo, my support is transferred to the lift chair.

In the seventh photo, I have begun the turn to sit in the chair. The eighth photo shows the last support from the scooter. The number of pictures and descriptions provided indicates how difficult and important this transfer was for me for a long time. One other thing to note is that the scooter seat is turned 90 degrees from the front. This reduces the risk of the scooter moving during the transfer because the force of getting up is 90 degrees from the wheel direction.

Seat Assist

When away from your house, your lift chair will not be there to help you get up. You will need to find other solutions. Initially,

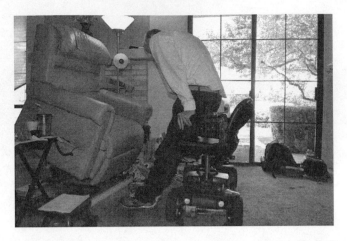

Scooter to lift chair #4, knees hyper-flexed backward (photograph by Taylor Bland).

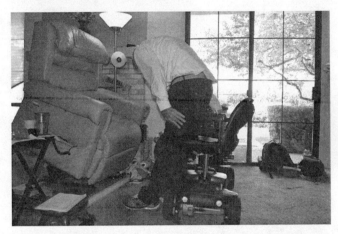

Scooter to lift chair #5, feet under shoulders (photograph by Taylor Bland).

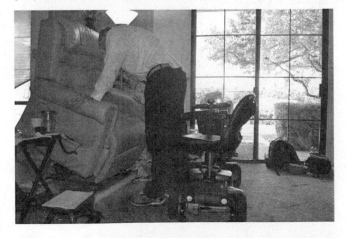

Scooter to lift chair #6, support transferred to lift chair (photograph by Taylor Bland).

you will be able to get up if a chair with arms is available. When you are at a restaurant or elsewhere where there aren't any armchairs, someone will have to help you get up. As I noted earlier, lifting on the back of your belt is an effective way for people to assist you. That is how people assisted me.

In the Blackhawk Plaza discussed in Chapter 4, there were three restaurants that I visited frequently. They had no chairs with the needed arms, but fortunately, the plaza did. These restaurants commandeered some and kept them available for me; one even put my name on one.

To maintain your independence longer, you will want to avoid constantly relying on other people to help you up. For your home, a Carex Uplift Premium Power Seat Assist is available to help you at your

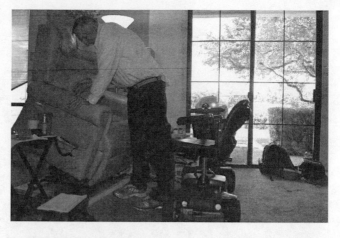

Scooter to lift chair #7, turning to sit in chair (photograph by Taylor Bland).

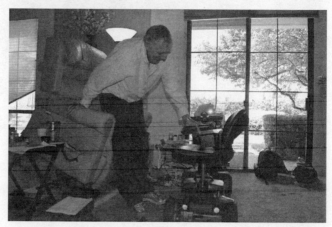

Scooter to lift chair #8, last support from scooter (photograph by Taylor Bland).

kitchen table or anywhere there is a power outlet. I wanted something that was not electrically operated so I could use it anywhere. I found my solution to be Carex Upeasy Seat Assist Plus.* I purchased one in March of 2015 from Amazon. A picture of mine on a patio chair is shown on the next page.

There are two versions based on your weight. Each version has multiple settings that change the lift strength desired. I found these so useful that I bought several. They fold down and can be easily transported wherever you go. I have used them on chairs, couches, cushioned armchairs, etc. I was surprised how few people knew about them, at least at that time. Frequently people came up to me at restaurants wanting to know what the device was and how they could buy one for a relative or friend. Even doctors expressed interest. My neurologist looked it up and pasted the website into her computer.

---

* These products can be bought on Amazon and other websites.

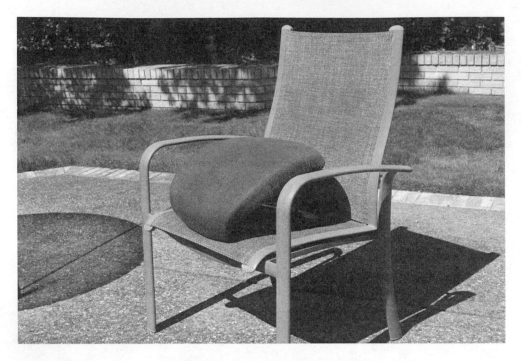

Seat assist (photograph by the author).

I found that when using the seat you should set the lift strength a little higher than recommended. If you do that, when you start to sit, there will be a little resistance. Then the seat assist will collapse down flat to a comfortable position. To get up, just lean forward and push down slightly with your arms on the chair.

Two notes of caution are warranted. Do not reach down to pick up anything on the floor. The weight transfer will tell the Seat Assist to get you up and it could eject you. Once it started to eject me, so I immediately shifted my weight back. The other concern was the occasional slippage of the Seat Assist on the chair. There is a thin layer of rubber on the bottom of the Seat Assist, but it doesn't cover the entire bottom. For most situations, that is adequate, but on some surfaces, such as metal, the seat assist could slip. This may not be a concern for most people, but because I used the Seat Assist so often, I bought a piece of thick rubber, cut it to the size of the bottom of the Seat Assist, and glued it on. I never had an issue with slippage again.

Walker

When I started using a walker, I no longer needed a chair with arms to get up. I didn't need a chair at all. I would sit on the walker seat and move in close to the table. I could push up on one of the relatively high arms with one hand and the walker's back support with the other to get up.

It is easy to transfer from a walker to any other device because you are already standing. First, face the walker in the opposite direction and then back up to your destination, whether to a lift chair, bed, toilet, table, etc.

Transferring Between the Scooter and the Wheelchair

I use both the scooter and the wheelchair in the house. Depending on what I plan to do that day, one device might be better than the other to accomplish those tasks. In many cases, I use one device for a few hours and then change to the other. Transferring between devices simply involves placing them beside each other at the appropriate distance and then adjusting the height and tilt of the wheelchair.

Transferring to and from the Bed

In the chapter on the walker, I mentioned that my walker is in daily use. I get up from the bed onto the walker. From there, I pivot and transfer to my mobility device, initially the scooter and later the wheelchair.

Getting Up from the Bed

As your muscles weaken, it becomes difficult to get up from a bed. I got to the point where I had to use enormous force to accomplish this. That amount of force created the possibility of my feet slipping, which could lead to a fall. Even though I had carpet in the bedroom, I still slipped at times. Hospital socks that have non-slip surfaces helped with the slippage issue but I knew I needed a better solution.

I was dealing with a company that works exclusively with disabled people. They sell medical equipment and also are a contractor that implements home modifications. Their recommendation was a balance pole. The pole went from the floor to the ceiling and had a few arms that stuck out horizontally from the pole. The idea is that you can grab the pole or an arm on the pole and pull yourself up. Different manufacturers call them a balance pole, security pole, transfer pole, or a floor to the ceiling grab bar. Unfortunately, it didn't work for me as I have to push straight down or pull straight down to get up. I returned the balance pole, but one might work for you.

The need for a better solution became very clear when I fell getting off a bed while at a family reunion in Tennessee. The bed wasn't high enough for the leverage I needed, so I pulled on a bedpost with one hand while pushing down on the bed with the other. My weakened hands slipped. I fell backward, my head missing a raised brick fireplace by inches which would have caused a devastating injury. As it was, it required a trip to the local hospital because of the injuries I had sustained.

The answer was purchasing low-cost bed risers. If I am traveling, I find out how many bedposts the bed has, the height from the floor to the top of the bed, and the bed legs' shape and size. I buy bed risers that will raise the bed to the height I need. In my case, the needed height is about 31", making the top of the bed level with my mid-thigh. I am 6'3" tall so that is one way to guess the height you need. It is very important to get the correct height. Raising the bed height to your mid-thigh might work but the required height depends on your strength.

Some hotels have ADA approved beds that should be high enough for most people. If its maximum height isn't 31", I bring short bed risers just in case. Make sure the bed legs will fit into the depression in the bed risers so it can't slip off. A set of four Slipstick 2" bed risers costs about $11. I bought these for a trip where the hotel had an ADA approved bed that had a maximum height of 29.5". For my home, I purchased two sets of eight Define Essentials multi-height bed risers that adjust to 8, 5 or 3" heights. Each set costs about $15.* A picture of the bed risers on my bed set at the 5" height is shown below.

The bed risers worked very well until July 2020 when I experienced more strength decline. I had been struggling to get up from the bed for some time. One morning as I was applying maximum force to get up, a foot slipped, and I fell hard from my elevated bed. A severe back injury was the most significant among several injuries I sustained. The pain affected my ability to care for my wife, Jodie, and myself.

I was lucky! Many worse outcomes were possible, particularly for my ability to be a caregiver. After that, I was terrified every time I needed to get up from the bed. As has been my practice, I started developing safer near-term methods for dressing, undressing, and getting up from the bed, while I searched for a long-term solution.

The 31" distance from the floor to the sleeping surface was no longer sufficient. I had the capability of raising the bed higher, but that raised other concerns. The stability of taller bed risers was one. Losing the ability to reach things on the floor while lying on the bed was another. But I had a related problem. In my increasingly weakened state, it was getting very tough to get into a sitting position before getting up. After the fall, it was also excruciating.

(The following discussion on electric beds was

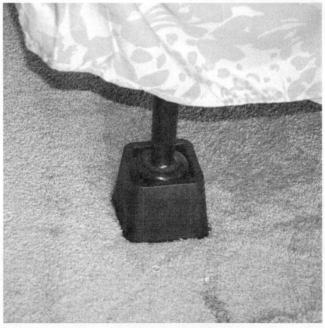

Bed riser (photograph by the author).

---

* The bed risers mentioned above can be purchased at Amazon and other websites.

added after we moved to a senior living facility in Phoenix and I had finished the first draft of this book.)

As I always try to look ahead, I knew that I might need a fully electric hospital bed someday but had not yet researched them. It seemed that a hospital bed could solve multiple problems. The bed could be lowered to make it easy to get into bed and to reach things on the floor. It could be raised above the 31" level to allow me to get up safely. The ability to raise the head end could help me get into a sitting position before getting out of bed and when reading in bed.

That was the theory! But after some research, I couldn't find any beds that could raise the sleeping surface, including the mattress, above 31"; most didn't go that high. I assumed that I could buy a deeper mattress but found that a 6" deep mattress was the best they could offer. It might be that deeper mattresses cause issues with articulating beds. I would research that later, if necessary.

I started by calling Invacare because I was familiar with that company. They gave me three nearby dealers. None of them sold their beds; one wasn't even located in the area. Through an Internet search, I found a local firm, Southwest Medical, that sold Invacare and Joerns beds. I eliminated Invacare because their maximum width was 36". Due to my size and the way I sleep, I thought that would be insufficient. The Joerns' beds had a maximum width of 42", which was not ideal either.

After more research, I found Preferred Health Choice (PHC), an Internet-based firm. They sell Tuffcare Full-Electric beds with widths of 48, 54, and 60". I bought the 54" model in early July 2020 for $4,645, including the 6" mattress. When I purchased it, PHC told me that the maximum height would be 32". I thought that would be a temporary solution because that would be an inch higher before I sat on the bed. My mattress is older and would sag more than a new 6" mattress so I would gain several inches. I planned to replace Tuff's 6" casters with 8" casters to increase the height. As I was not able to get specific enough information to order them to arrive before the bed, I elected to see whether they were needed immediately.

The bed arrived quickly and was assembled by the facility's maintenance personnel the same day. That was very fortunate because I had the strength to get up only once at night, and the danger of doing that was so dangerous it terrified me. That wasn't the only good news. When I measured the maximum height, it was 34", 3" higher than my bed, not counting the mattress sag difference. Following are pictures showing the maximum and minimum bed heights.

In just a couple of days, I found that several heights worked best for different needs. I don't yet need the maximum height to get up safely, thus extending the time until I need larger casters or an alternate method to gain elevation. With the weakness and pain I have, I use a reacher to assist me when dressing and undressing* at another elevation. To increase my safety when getting up in the

---

* The vertical stud at the end of the reacher can be used to push pants, socks and shoes off your legs and feet when your feet are slightly above ground level. It can also drag things close to you that are on the floor. The grabber can pick up clothing from any location you can reach and can help pull pants up your legs.

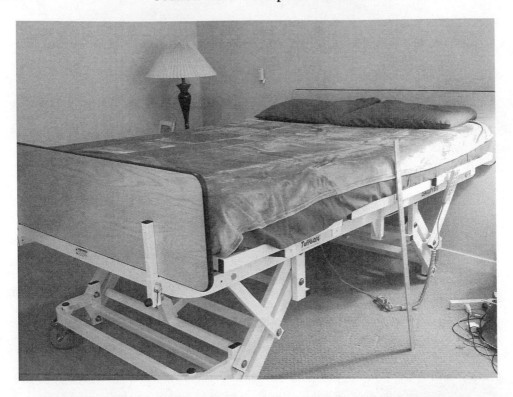

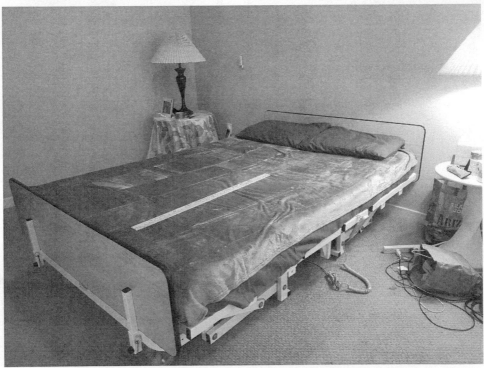

Top: Bed in maximum height position. *Bottom:* Bed in minimum height position (photographs by the author).

middle of the night, I found that an elevation slightly above the floor allows me to push my bare feet into my loosely tied shoes, which are on the floor. At that elevation, I don't have to lift my legs, allowing me to avoid some pain. Then I can push down with my legs to get my feet into the shoes. With the shoes on, I don't have to worry about slippage, which caused the fall that led to purchasing this bed.

I use two elevations to get into bed. A slightly lower height than the one I use to stand up from the bed is necessary to sit down on it. The lowest possible height is used when I pull my legs onto the bed. I avoid almost all the pain I experienced getting my legs on my old bed at the lowest height.

The bed has other capabilities, e.g., both the head end and the foot end can be elevated. My feet swell because I can't walk. It helps to raise my feet above the level of my heart at night to reduce the swelling. The bed has backup batteries and a light at the bottom of the bed, making the bed functional in power outages.

If your issues differ from mine, any of the options I considered could work for you.

Transferring to and from the toilet is covered in the next chapter, Handicap Toilet Progression.

14

Handicap Toilet Progression

"The spectacular is always preceded by a long period of unspectacular preparation."
—Kenneth McFarland, quoted in "Youth Should Be Told Truths,"
The Decatur [Illinois] *Daily Review*, October 13, 1944

When dealing with a progressive disease affecting your muscles, you will soon find that the ability to use a standard toilet has become impossible. The challenges associated with toiletry mirror those of getting up from chairs. New solutions are needed when what had been working no longer does. The typical first step is a new toilet with a higher seat. As your strength declines further, a raised toilet seat with arms that fits on top of the toilet bowl is a helpful choice. The raised arms allow you to push down to assist in standing. If you search: "Raised toilet seat with arms," you will find many choices. These devices are very useful when traveling and they are easy to pack. I purchased the Carex E-Z Lock Raised Toilet Seat with Handles.* A picture of mine is shown here.

When these solutions no longer work, commodes that sit on the floor and rise above the toilet seat are the next step. My first commode was a Drive Medical Steel Folding Bedside Commode. It was both helpful and cost-effective at $30 to $40.

A picture of the Drive Medical Commode is shown on the following page.

During a trip to Cornwall, England I found a much better option. Our B&B had an Etac

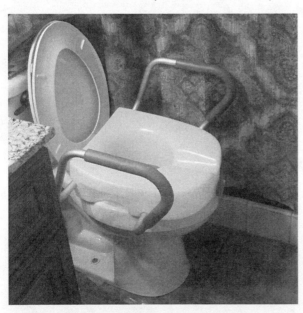

Raised toilet seat (photograph by Mike Reed).

---

* You can find that model for about $40 by searching with the description above on multiple sites.

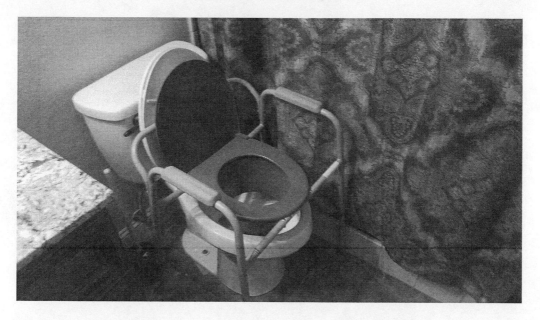

Drive medical commode (photograph by Lisa Reed).

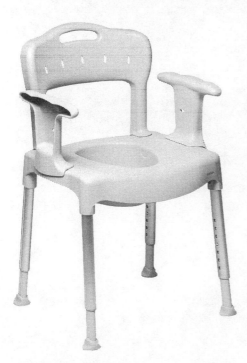

Swift Commode chair* and I purchased one when we returned home. See the picture on the left.

Eventually, my needs changed again. I needed a chair that could raise the seat even higher and be packed in a suitcase. I found one made by Nuprodx Mobility.[1] The company was very accommodating and modified the design to make it adjustable to higher levels than was possible with its original model. This worked well on trips.

The picture on the following page shows the model I bought, MC4000TX, as well as the travel case. While I used it only as a commode, it could also be used for showering when there is someone who can move you in and out of the shower.

I still have this commode for travel, but it is no longer in use at home.† I now have a shower chair with wheelchair wheels that I use for both toiletry and showering. I will describe that commode in the next chapter.

Etac Swift Commode chair (photograph by Joanna Goldberg of Etac AB).

---

* You can find that model for about $170 by searching with the description above.
† When we moved to a senior living facility in Phoenix, it was used again as a commode.

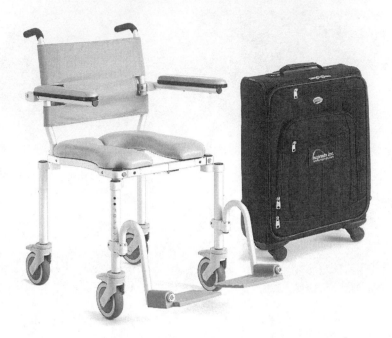

Nuprodx commode and case (photograph by permission of Nuprodx).

If you are at the initial stages of your disease progression, you may want to skip some steps I went through and immediately purchase two commodes, one for the home and one for the road, which will meet your needs in the foreseeable future.

The next chapter, Showering Safely, describes the process I went through to find a safe showering method that I could accomplish without assistance.

15

Showering Safely

"Achievement is talent plus preparation."
—Malcolm Gladwell, in *Outliers: The Story of Success* (2008)

The typical style of this book is to discuss options, followed by the decisions I made and the rationale behind those decisions. This chapter is more about the process I went through to make a viable decision to solve my need to shower independently and safely. Your situation may be different from mine, but there may be elements of my decision process that would be of value to you.

Considering my condition, the risk I was taking of falling when showering was unacceptable. Even when I needed to use a mobility device to go anywhere, I was still taking stand-up showers. Making matters even worse, my shower stall had a curb-height entrance that I had to step over. I used the walker to get to the shower entrance and then stepped into the shower. From the experience of several trips to the emergency room from falls unrelated to showering, I had learned that I had to either push straight down or hold onto something directly above me to avoid falling when entering the shower. Reaching straight out for support would not work because my knees would collapse. Using a multiple-step process, I reached up with one hand and held on to the top of the glass entrance panel. Then as I stepped into the shower, I pushed down with the other hand on the faucet until I was in the shower. After that, I relied on both legs being hyper-extended backward to avoid falling. Getting out was equally risky. It sounds crazy even writing this! If I had fallen, it could have been catastrophic. The inside of the shower was a very constrained, tight space. Getting my legs and arms out of the way of serious harm would have been impossible, and there was a head injury risk. Family and friends continually urged me to find a safer way to shower which finally motivated me to find a better solution.

The reason for my procrastination was that I didn't like my options. If I wanted to be independent, I had to be able to shower any time without help. This eliminated many good possibilities many others might choose such as having a caregiver help you get in and out of the shower.

Our master bathroom has two rooms. The main room contains sinks, cabinets and a sunken tub. The shower room includes the toilet, shower stall, and a small closet. The lowest cost and fastest to implement option was to buy a slide

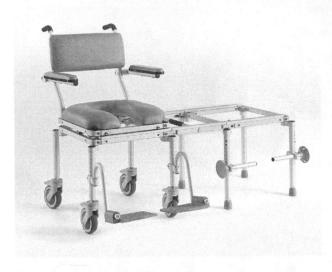

Nuprodx tub slider system (photograph by permission of Nuprodx).

transfer system. This solution would involve a specialized commode that would sit over the toilet. By placing a companion device in the shower and connecting them with transfer arms, the seat can slide from the toilet into the shower. It is also possible to go over a tub edge or a shower curb. A picture of one solution found on Nuprodx.com is shown above. That website also has a video of the system in use with the aid of a caregiver.[*]

The slide transfer option was not chosen because of certain limitations: my toilet was not as close to the shower as desired for this system; it required the installation of a device in the shower which would have to be removed each time Jodie wished to shower; and I would have had to install and remove the connecting arms each time I showered. These limitations caused me to look for another solution. However, many readers could find this to be their best option.

A different approach, which I finally chose, was to construct a zero-threshold shower, either in place of the present shower or in the larger main room of the master bathroom. I was advised by family and friends, some of whom have engineering degrees, two contractors, and the Nuprodx president.

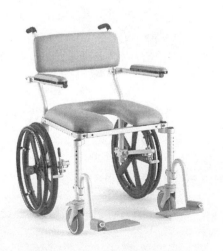

Nuprodx toilet/shower chair (photograph by permission of Nuprodx).

Initially, most advisors believed that the shower room was too small to hold a zero-threshold shower. That left what would be a major, costly and unsightly modification of the master bathroom's main room. The sunken tub would have to be removed and some windows

---

[*] https://youtu.be/R5-oHvt-a3s.

would be blocked. This approach could adversely impact the home's resale value. The advantage was there would be room for the large zero-threshold shower. This was the option advocated by most people, particularly my family who wanted what was best for me and cared much less about other factors.

I wanted to see whether it was possible to modify the shower room because of the major disadvantages of modifying the main room. The president of Nuprodx was the strongest proponent of this option. The concept was to remove the small closet and extend the shower into that area. I would also have to purchase a new toilet/shower chair. However, that would be a necessary purchase regardless of where I built the new shower. A picture of the chair I was considering is shown at the bottom of the previous page.

But would widening the shower provide enough room to maneuver the toilet/shower chair to and from the toilet and the enlarged shower?

I knew Tim Heck, my contractor, had built mock-ups of potential room changes for George Homolka, one of my friends. I thought a mock-up would be the best way to make an informed decision and asked Tim to construct a mock-up of the modified room on my driveway to perform a dry run.

Tim built the mock-up using sheetrock for walls, a plywood piece to show the toilet space and tape to show the expected shower floor. Nuprodx, the equipment supplier, brought the toilet/shower chair, which would allow me to dry run the process.

Following are some pictures of the mock-up taken by David Gaskell, president of Nuprodx.

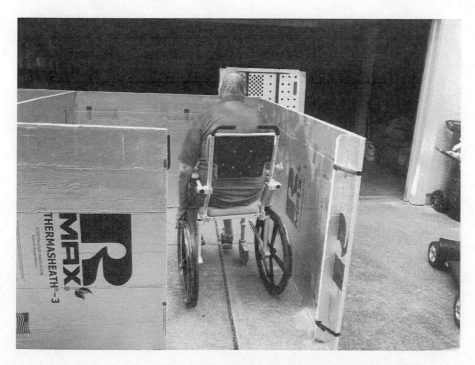

Entering mock-up shower room (photograph by David Gaskell).

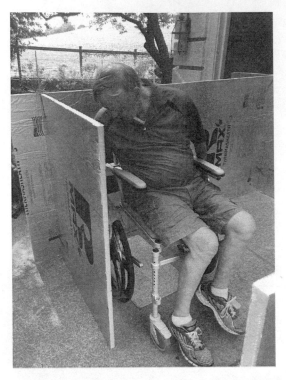

Backed up over mock-up toilet (photograph by David Gaskell).

The two pictures demonstrate that I could enter the shower room and back over the toilet (modeled as plywood cut to the toilet size).

The picture below shows that I could then maneuver into the shower (outlined in tape on the floor).

The pictures on the following page show the original and modified shower rooms.

We also built a platform underneath the toilet to reduce the amount of splashing caused by the toilet chair being so far above the standard toilet height.

Again, Nuprodx customized the toilet/shower chair to allow extra height on the legs. I found one significant drawback with the portable commode. It was difficult to clean after using the toilet because of the stabilizing bar right under the seat's front. This was necessary for

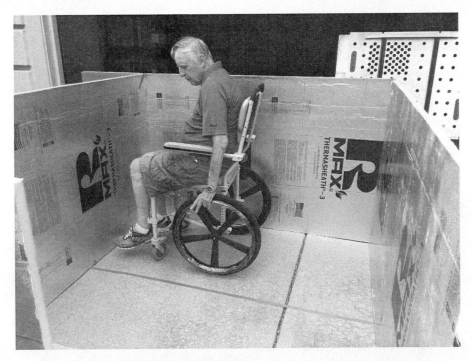

In the mock-up shower (photograph by David Gaskell).

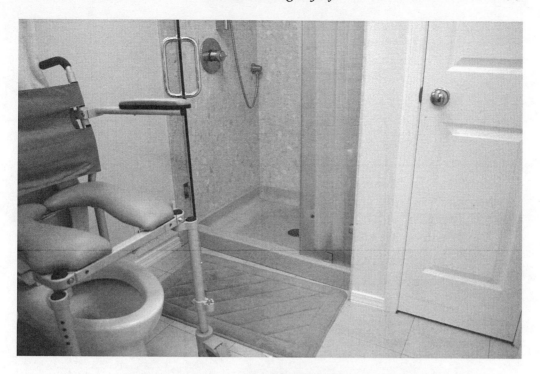

Original shower room (photograph by the author).

the portable toilet chair to fit in a suitcase.

When I purchased the toilet/shower chair, I asked them to modify the design and lower that bar to facilitate cleaning. They changed the design; it is now the standard for their product.

You can see the chair's lowered front bar and the toilet platform in the picture on the next page.

After modifying the shower room and purchasing the chair, I safely used both the toilet and shower. I would not have been willing to take the risk of modifying the shower room without the confirmation provided by the mock-up. If you have a significant decision concerning a remodeling project and are unsure of its viability, consider first getting a mock-up made.

I had excellent cooperation

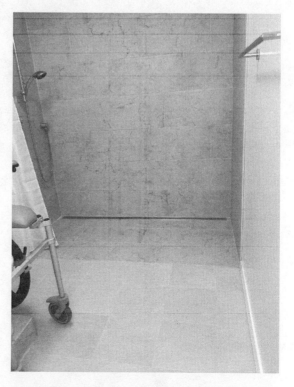

Reconstructed shower room (photograph by the author).

from Nuprodx. I feel one reason this level of cooperation was possible is that the owner is disabled himself. My understanding is that he started designing solutions for himself, then created Nuprodx to market his concepts. The fact that the company is located locally and the president lives in my town were also factors. However, I believe they are more flexible in accommodating their customers' needs than many other firms.

I learned about Nuprodx from the firm that sold me the Nuprodx travel commode and the lifts in my house, and learned about my contractor from one of my golf friends years ago. The contacts I had developed through friends and from seeking local expertise to solve earlier problems had helped me find the ideal

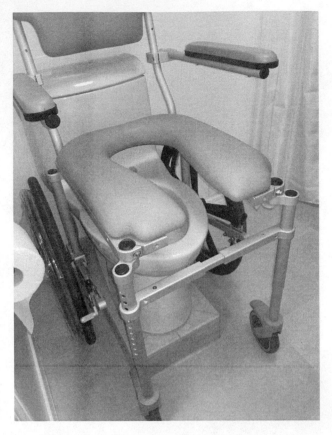

Toilet/shower chair and pedestal (photograph by the author).

solution in this case and will be helpful for future challenges. Going to support groups, networking with friends and business associates, and searching for local expertise are all ways that can lead to better solutions for the challenges you will face.

The next chapter discusses the various options for acquiring food if your condition or circumstances make this difficult.

16

Food and Shopping

"Only someone who is well prepared has the opportunity to improvise."

—Ingmar Bergman

When neither Jodie nor I could drive, keeping sufficient food on hand was challenging. Because of her cognitive issues, I stopped Jodie from cooking meals for safety reasons. If anything dangerous happened when she was using the stove, it would take too long for me to get up from the lift chair, onto the wheelchair and into the kitchen to help. Also, my physical limitations might limit my ability to solve the problem. Several scares made that decision a necessity. As a result, few meals are made at home. I don't want Jodie to see me cooking. It might cause her to want to cook as well; I only do it when we have no other option.

Fortunately, there are now many ways to acquire food. Groceries and almost everything else needed can be purchased through Amazon. Many grocery stores like Safeway, Fresh Foods, and Costco deliver. Some restaurants, including most pizza restaurants, deliver meals as well.

I use Safeway and Costco for bulk deliveries. I used to order about once a week from Costco, but Joel, one of my golf friends, delivers us food from Costco when he is shopping there about every ten days, so we don't need a Costco delivery very often now.

If you have the right timing, you can get free delivery, a $10 to $20 discount, and special prices for items you buy in large quantities from Safeway. It still costs more than shopping in the stores where better offers and special deals exist, but for us, delivery is a much more effective way to acquire food.

Many services will pick up food from restaurants and deliver it to your door. DoorDash, Uber Eats, Instacart, Grubhub, Seamless, Postmates, Gopuff, Delivery.com, and Eat24 are some of the well-known ones. By checking their websites, you can determine if they deliver from restaurants you like and what they charge. We use DoorDash about once a week. Getting food this way is great for last-minute decisions. If you order a few times a month, it is worth joining Dash-Pass. It costs $10/month but saves you $3 to $5 per order.

Another option is using Munchery, Home Chef, HelloFresh, Plated, and many other firms that prepare full meal kits. These may work for you. As we don't need full meals, and they usually have to be heated, we don't use this service.

We use Paratransit about once a week to get to restaurants, allowing us to eat a meal and then bring home enough food for one or more meals. The biggest benefit is that of getting out of the house to enjoy life. We also always go to a grocery store like Trader Joe's, Draeger's or Safeway to stock up on food when we go out to eat. Paratransit only allows three bags of groceries, so larger orders have to be placed with Costco, Safeway or other supermarkets that deliver. There are additional restrictions on what Paratransit will transport for you. For example, Coca-Cola's cases are too heavy and bulky to ask drivers to carry them.

I must be on a gluten-free diet* because I have Celiac disease.† That complicates my meal choices. I can't eat bread, pasta, pizza, most soups, and many other things unless they are made gluten-free. It is not always easy to know if there is gluten in the food you eat, particularly at restaurants. If you need this particular diet, read labels, look for gluten-free selections available on the menu, and ask questions. Some grocery stores have gluten-free sections.

Even small amounts can cause the body to mount an immune response that attacks the small intestine. These attacks lead to damage to the villi, small finger-like projections lining the small intestine that promote nutrient absorption. When the villi become damaged, nutrients cannot be adequately absorbed into the body. For more information on Celiac disease, visit Celiac.org.[1] For a comprehensive list of sources and foods that contain gluten, visit drperlmutter.com.[2]

The next chapter offers suggestions for solving problems you may face daily.

---

* Gluten is a protein found in wheat, rye, and barley.
† Celiac disease is an autoimmune disease where ingestion of gluten leads to damage in the small intestine. It is estimated to affect 1 in 100 people worldwide and 1 in 10 people who are a first-degree relative of someone with Celiac disease, i.e, parent, child, or sibling. Two and a half million Americans are undiagnosed and are at risk for long-term health complications.

17

Solutions to Daily Issues

"A clever person solves a problem. A wise person avoids it."
—Albert Einstein

One of the most useful items I found for people with mobility issues is a reacher, aka a grabber. I have three of them, one 24 inches and two 32 inches long. I use them multiple times every day. There are many options that you will find via a web search. A picture of one of my 32" reachers is shown below.[*]

You can reach a distance of nine feet or more with a 32" reacher by leaning forward. I keep one of them near my bed and one near my lift chair. As you can see from the picture, the reacher has a pistol grip and a claw that allows you to pick up large items like a pair of slacks or small things like a penny. It has a magnetic end as well which is occasionally useful. The vertical projection on the claw end can be used to drag things to you by turning the reacher upside down.

Two other very useful items are the clothing stick and a long shoehorn. Examples are pictured on the next page.

I am still able to dress but have trouble buttoning things.[†] I have Jodie pre-button shirts and leave the top button unbuttoned. That way I can pull them over my head instead of buttoning them. When I need to button something, I use a button hook. They can be found on Amazon and work well. The Vive Button Hook-Zipper Pull Helper is a good choice.

Putting on socks can be a challenge but there are sock aids that can solve that

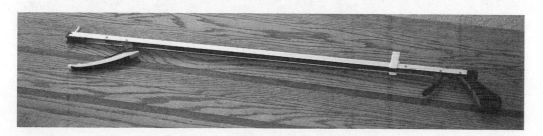

Reacher or grabber (photograph by the author).

---

[*] The picture shows one of the RMS 2-Pack 32" Long Grabber/Reachers purchased on Amazon.
[†] Issues with buttoning are mentioned specifically as an IBM symptom by Cleveland Clinic.

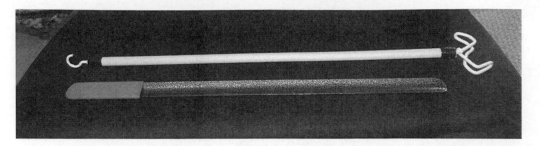

Clothing stick and long shoehorn (photograph by Maylina Hutchins).

problem. The first one I tried didn't work. Later I found one that used more flexible material that did work.

By placing my clothing and shoes near my bed, I can sit on the edge of my bed in the morning and retrieve everything I need to get dressed with a reacher. This saves the time and energy that it takes to get up, transfer to my wheelchair, get my clothes, and then reverse the process to go back to bed to get dressed. I accomplish this by having clean underwear and at least the pair of pants that I'm going to wear the next day close to my bed within the range of the reacher. It isn't necessary to have a shirt nearby because that can be put on while in your mobility device. I have a bag of socks and my shoes on the floor which my reacher can also grab. The reacher can also be used to pick up dropped items like a watch, pencil, etc.

Like many other chapters in this book, my circumstances changed after writing this chapter. I could no longer put on my underpants because I couldn't lift my left leg high enough. I was able to solve the problem with the reacher. By leaving the underpants on the floor with one leg inserted, the reacher could grab the underpants, open them up so the second leg could be inserted without lifting it much, and then pull up the underpants until I could reach them.

The reacher is similarly useful when I am in my lift chair. I drop a lot of things with my weak hands. I retrieve them with the reacher. Occasionally, things fall in other parts of the house in narrow spaces that the reacher can recover. One word of caution, however. If you are picking up something heavy, you will be using a significant amount of force. Make sure that you are not pulling up in the direction of your face. If the item slips off the reacher, the reacher could come back and hit your face. I don't have to tell you how I know this.

I have a few other suggestions for inexpensive items that can improve your life. In the photo on the opposite page, from left to right are pictured some foam grip tubing on a spoon, a screw-top glass with a bent straw and two rubber grippers.

The foam grip tubing was given to me by a physical therapist because he knew I had weak hands. It gives you something larger, round, and flexible to hold. That foam grip tubing could be cut in half lengthwise and used for two pieces of silverware. This tubing can be used on other items like a toothbrush, a shaver, etc. Currently, I don't need this but I may someday. If you have difficulty holding silverware or other things, you might want to consider buying foam grip tubing. Just search for "foam grip tubing." If you search for handicap silverware, you will find many pre-made handicap silverware options. It is even possible to have a device that attaches to your hand that will allow you to change from a spoon to a fork. See Therafin—Universal Feeding Cuff "Fork and Spoon Holder" as an example.

Because of the weakness of my hands, I drop several items each day. This is a real problem when the item is a glass of liquid. The screw-top plastic container, top, and straw pictured in the middle of the picture below[*] solved 95 percent of the problem for me. I buy bent straws separately because it is easier for me to drink with them than the straight straws that come with the containers. If you look carefully at the bottom of the straw, you will see an enlarged diameter that prevents the straw from coming out if the glass falls. You can even pick up the glass by the straw. It is best to buy these at a store together because the enlarged bottom has to be bigger than the lid hole.

The rubber grippers on the right side of the picture are essential to my independent living. Without them, I wouldn't be able to open a bottle of water, a carton of milk, a plastic bottle of orange juice, a jar of pickles, etc. For that reason, I have several of them and use them daily. Sometimes the grippers are essential but not enough. For glass jars with metal tops, I sometimes have to bang on the lid with a butter knife around the lid before I use the gripper to get it open. The

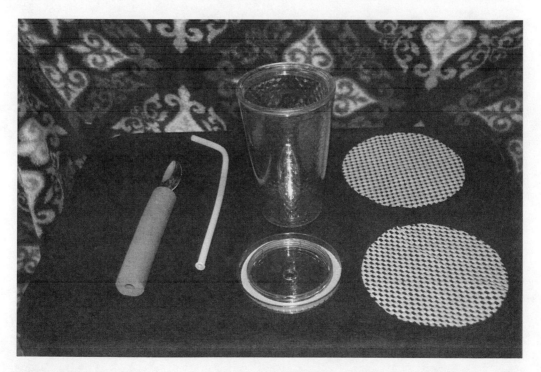

Silverware holder, bent straw, screw-top glass and rubber grippers (photograph by Maylina Hutchins).

---

[*] *Cupture Beehive Orange/Honey Color Insulated Double Wall Tumbler Cups—16 oz.* They come with straight straws.

reason this works is that the contents were sealed at high temperatures which creates a vacuum in the jar when the contents cool. Banging the lid helps reduce the vacuum.

When my friend, Bill Huber, who reviewed my chapters and suggested edits, read the first draft of this chapter, he asked whether cups with handles would be helpful. It reminded me that in the early stages of my muscle weakness, I used cups with handles. As I got weaker, however, the cup and contents' weight would sometimes cause my wrist to collapse and dump the contents. I realized that a cup with handles that had a screw-top and straw would be a great solution. As a result of an Internet search, I found some Mason jar tumblers with a lid and straw. I immediately bought two of them and I recommend them to anyone with hand and wrist weakness. They are 20-ounce containers pictured below.

The tumblers come with straight straws but my bent straws fit reasonably well.

Search for "Cupture 2 Vintage Blue Mason Jar Tumbler Mug with Stainless Steel Lid and Straw–20 oz" on Amazon or elsewhere to find them.

This is the last chapter of the Independent Life section of the book. The next two sections address ways to achieve vehicle mobility when using a motorized scooter or wheelchair.

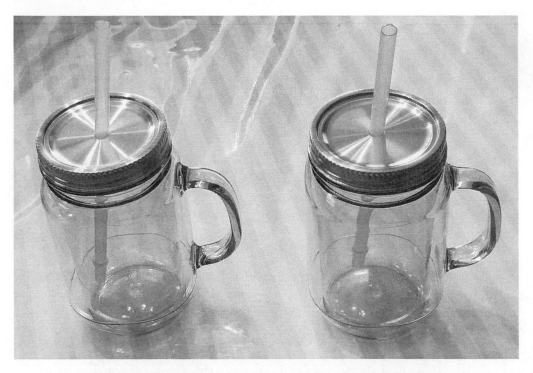

Tumblers with screw tops and straws (photograph by the author).

Vehicle Mobility

"Be the kind of person who dares to face life's challenges and overcome them rather than dodging them."
— Roy T. Bennett, *The Light in the Heart*

This section describes the methods we used for vehicle transportation once I had to use a motorized mobility device because I could no longer walk or safely use a walker. Initially, I used a motorized scooter and later a wheelchair. While I was using a scooter, I had to find a way to travel using my SUV. That is the subject of Chapter 18 and was my mode of transportation while I could drive and afterward when someone was available to drive me.

We had to use public transportation when no one could drive me, and later when my mobility device was a motorized wheelchair. That is the subject of Chapter 19.

18

Vehicle Adaptation for a Motorized Scooter

"Luck is what happens when preparation meets opportunity."
—Seneca

While I still had sufficient strength to drive, I could continue to use my sport utility vehicle (SUV) to get wherever I wanted. It was simply a matter of putting my cane, and later my fold-up walker, into the back seat. My mobility became a more complicated issue in mid–September 2016. My strength weakened to the point where I needed to have a motorized scooter outside the house. I had paid a local medical equipment dealer $1,953 for a Pride Go-Go Sport 4-Wheel scooter. As I couldn't take it apart to put it into the SUV,* I had to have another way to transport the scooter.

The solution to this problem was to install a platform on the back of the SUV. Pride Mobility Products Corporation, the manufacturer of my scooter, sells a platform that can be installed on a hitch on the back of the vehicle and connected to the electrical system in the SUV. A picture of my SUV with the scooter lift on the back is shown here.

The platform is vertical when not in use. Vision through the back window is restricted somewhat, but there are holes in

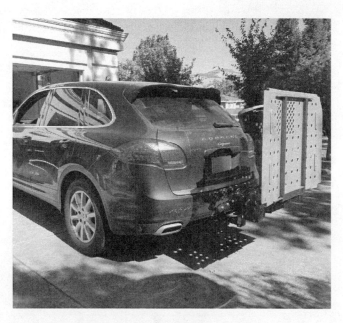

Scooter lift unloaded (photograph by the author).

* My son could do this when I visited him but no one could do it on a daily basis for me.

the platform so you can see sufficiently well. Visibility with the scooter loaded is slightly better because the platform rises after the scooter is loaded from the down position and slightly rotates toward the car as it rises, but it doesn't rise all the way up.

One annoying thing about having a platform on the back of the vehicle is the car senses that there is something behind it, so it makes a warning sound to alert you. Fortunately, the alarm turns off reasonably quickly. My SUV has a rearview camera to enable me to check that there are no obstructions behind me when I am backing up.

If you buy just the platform, it is impossible to open the liftgate, but I purchased the Pride Outlander Full Platform[*] and the Swing-Away Adapter.[†] The Swing-Away Adapter allows access to the rear cargo area as shown below.

The platform can be swung out of the way by pulling out a pin and lifting a handle. The scooter should not be on the platform when you use the Swing-Away Adapter as it is not designed for that extra weight.

I didn't purchase the platform from a local medical equipment dealer, who would have subcontracted the electrical work to U–Haul or some other company.

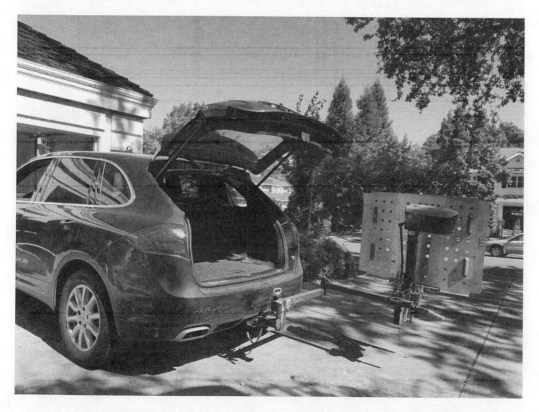

Scooter lift swung away for trunk access (photograph by the author).

---

[*] The Outlander platform can be found at: https://www.pridemobility.com/p/outlander.
[†] The swing-away adapter and other accessories can be found at https://www.pridemobility.com/p/outlander/accessories.

Instead, I purchased the platform from Spinlife.com and convinced U-Haul that installing the lifts could be a new business for them. They agreed, so I had the equipment sent directly to them for installation. This approach resulted in significant cost savings. I paid Spinlife $2,150 for the platform and U-Haul $365 for the hitch plus $236 for the platform installation, wiring, and tail-light converter.

In the picture below, to load the scooter, you lower the platform from the vertical position flat on the ground. The scooter can then be driven onto the platform. Note in the photo below that the left wheels (as viewed by the scooter driver) are over the left holes.

When the platform is lifted with the scooter on it, the system realizes it has a load. As it rises, a hold-down device pivots down and presses against the scooter's base to secure it. There was no instruction from the manufacturer that indicated that it was critical that the hold-down device press down at the platform's center. It made sense to do that, however, so that was my practice. It was necessary to place the left wheels over the left holes to achieve the hold-down device's centering. I did a lot of driving, sometimes over rough roads in a national park using that procedure without incident. The picture on the next page shows the hold-down device centered.

I learned how important centering the hold-down device was when I loaded the scooter one time and realized that it wasn't quite in the middle of the scooter platform but was reasonably close. I didn't think that was crucial. I was only going

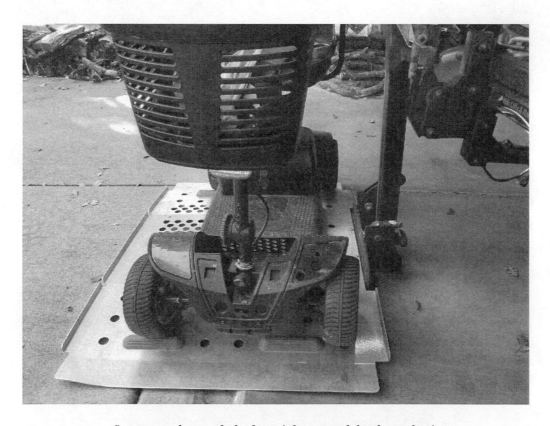

Scooter on lowered platform (photograph by the author).

to drive a short distance on a low-traffic road. When I got home, I went to take the scooter off the platform and found it wasn't there. Immediately, we turned around and retraced our route but found nothing.

Later I learned that a person came down the road shortly after we did and saw the scooter on the side of the road. He picked it up and took it home thinking his mother could use it for spare parts on her scooter. After a few days, he notified the police that he had it. He told them the owner could have it back if he could identify it. Since I had previously alerted the police, they called and I recovered it. The incident proved to me that I had to make sure the hold-down bar was centered. Otherwise, the scooter could shake off.

The scooter fell off a second time after I could no longer drive or load the scooter myself. My golf friend, John Wyatt, nearly always offered to drive me to our golf group lunches after they played so I could maintain those relationships. He had successfully loaded the scooter many times, but it came off again and separated into several pieces along the road in one such trip.

Afterward, John recalled that he had not completely centered the bar. Since we had been on our way to lunch with the rest of our golf group, we called them and they quickly came to our assistance. My friend, George Homolka, reassembled all the pieces and put the scooter back in working order with help from the others. We added a ratchet belt he had in his car to provide two ways to secure the

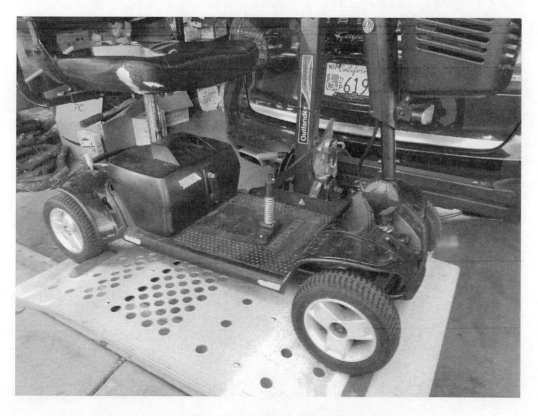

Scooter hold-down centered (photograph by the author).

scooter. I decided that it was too dangerous for other drivers who might run into scooter debris if it came off again. We used the ratchet belt every time after that and never had a problem again.

The picture below shows the hold-down device and the ratchet belt in place, safely securing the scooter to the scooter lift platform.

For quite a while, I could load the scooter myself and work my way to the driver's seat by leaning against the car. I put some suction cup handles like those sometimes used in showers on the side of my SUV to move between the lift and the driver's seat safely. By the end of May 2017, however, my legs weakened to the point where it was no longer safe for me to drive. I could no longer switch quickly from the gas pedal to the brake. I had been able to drive the way a race car driver would by putting my heel on the floor and rotating my foot from the gas to the brake. I knew it was no longer safe to drive when I attempted to rotate on my heel in an emergency. Muscle memory took over and did what came naturally after decades of driving; I lifted my foot off the gas pedal to hit the brake. My leg was not strong enough to do that and fell to the floor. I had to lift my leg with my hand to move it to the brake.

I got home using one foot on the gas and one on the brake, which caused a muscle cramp in my leg. I was relieved to get home and decided I would never drive again. Even if I never had another cramp, the risk of the foot slipping off the brake was too high. I sent a note on May 27, 2017, to friends and family telling

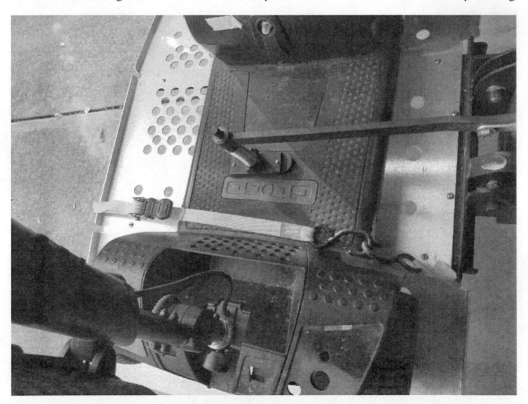

Scooter secured by hold-down and ratchet belt (photograph by the author).

them that I wasn't going to drive anymore. (It would be 30 months before I could drive again, this time using hand controls.)

At the time I stopped driving, Jodie was still able to drive. However, her memory had declined to the point where she was getting lost. She even got lost returning home from our town, though we had lived there for 32 years. When she got lost, she needed directions from me by phone. Unfortunately, she could not always use the phone to call me or to answer my calls.* Once I had to call the police and ask them to look for her. I was very concerned because she should have been at home. When I called her phone, a customer at Walgreens answered it. She had left it on the floor. In that instance, she eventually found her way home, but I decided that she could only drive when I was in the car.

Two months later, she was scheduled to be retested by the California Department of Motor Vehicles (DMV) on her birthday in late July. It was evident that she couldn't pass a written test, so we didn't go to the DMV. I was relieved that she lost her driver's license because she kept thinking that she could drive alone and I was afraid she might try it when I was out with friends.

For 30 months after that, the only way we could get around in a personal vehicle was when someone loaded my scooter on my SUV platform and drove us. As mentioned earlier, John Wyatt usually dove me to lunch with my former golf partners every week or so. When relatives or out-of-state friends visited us, they would drive us. When we visited with out-of-state families during the holidays, a family member would breakdown my scooter, put it in the trunk of their vehicle until we got to our destination, then reassemble it.† However, these occasions were infrequent so our vehicle mobility was minimal.

We needed a way to get to doctors' appointments, grocery stores, etc. Also, we wanted to get out to lunch, dinner or a movie to enjoy life. George Homolka told me about Paratransit which became our primary travel method for about two and a half years.

The next chapter describes how to use public transportation when you have a mobility device like a motorized scooter or wheelchair, which is how we had to travel most of the time until I learned to drive with hand controls.

---

* I had taken away her smart phone and replaced it with a flip phone but that was still a big challenge for her.

† It doesn't take very long to pull off the seat, pull off the battery pack and then fold the steering wheel column down.

19

Public Transport

Adapt or perish, now as ever, is Nature's inexorable imperative.
—H.G. Wells, in *Mind at the End of Its Tether* (1945)

Depending on your level of disability, there are many options for public transport. If you have the physical ability to fold a wheelchair or someone to do that for you, you will be able to use Uber, Lift, taxicabs, etc. The options are more limited when you have a motorized scooter or wheelchair. Over time, Uber and other companies will probably provide a service that can transport motorized mobility devices, but that is not available now, at least not where I live. Eventually, self-driving vehicles will be available, but it does not seem likely that they will be able to transport motorized scooters or wheelchairs.

As explained in the previous chapter, after July 2017, neither Jodie nor I could drive. Because I was dependent on either a motorized scooter or wheelchair, the only option for us was the Complementary Paratransit system.* I was able to get the paperwork needed to use that system approved that month by our neurologist. Jodie and I took our first trip in mid–July.

There is a good article on Paratransit and Complementary Paratransit on the National Aging and Disability Transportation Center website.[1] Here is a summary from their website:

> The Americans with Disabilities Act (ADA) requires public transit agencies that provide fixed-route service to provide "complementary paratransit" service to people with disabilities who cannot use the fixed-route bus or rail service because of a disability. The ADA regulations specifically define a population of customers who are entitled to this service as a civil right. The regulations also define minimum service characteristics that must be met for this service to be considered equivalent to the fixed-route service it is intended to complement.

While what I use is Complementary Paratransit, I will use the term "Paratransit" in this book. With Paratransit, a motorized mobility device can be lifted onto a bus. It is a valuable service that we used when going to doctor appointments, restaurants, grocery stores, etc. Check to see if your community has a Paratransit system that will transport disabled people. If so, obtain a doctor's recommendation and sign up.

---

* That was the case for over two years until September 2019 when I started driving a hand-controlled van.

Paratransit is inexpensive. Our total cost for two-plus years of use was less than $1,000. However, there are significant disadvantages associated with using it. Last-minute reservations are impossible because reservations must be made at least one day in advance. There is no service on Saturdays or Sundays when people want to go to dinner or a movie. This leaves you at home every weekend. They give you a 30-minute pickup window. While it is reasonable to have a 30-minute window, you have to plan for a pickup at any time during that window as well as arrivals outside that window. This can result in arriving at your destination too late or too early. If they pick you up from home late, you might not have enough time to do everything planned. This needs to be considered when making your reservations.

The service is deficient in many regards. When things go wrong with the transport's schedule, it is hard to get an update. You can't track your bus to see where it is or get an estimated arrival time without calling dispatch. Dispatch is so understaffed that they often put you on hold for an extended period. Without that information, you don't know whether the transport will be late and, if so, by how much. That means you can't make alternate plans or find out whether your appointment can be adjusted.

In one case, I had a critical appointment with a neurologist who was going to help get my wheelchair approved by Medicare. The bus was very late and Paratransit put me on hold to the point where it was impossible to get to the appointment in time using Paratransit. The neurologist's policy was to cancel the appointment and charge me. Luckily, my neighbor Steve Steen was home and rushed over to convey Jodie, the scooter and me to the appointment in my SUV. In another case, they were so late on the pickup from home that I couldn't possibly get done what I needed to accomplish. I reached them to try to reschedule the pickup time for the trip home, but they wouldn't reschedule it. I was told that they would try to get me home later. After hours of waiting, a Good Samaritan saw what was happening and helped us get into his truck. He broke down the scooter and drove us home. It has been my experience that many thoughtful people will go to great lengths to help disabled people.

Paratransit organizations sometimes have a mixture of both vans and busses to transport people. If you are using a motorized scooter, you will find that the vans are not suitable. I couldn't take a motorized scooter into a Paratransit van without having to ride with the scooter oriented perpendicular to the front of the vehicle. Because I could not get out of the scooter and into a chair, I had to ride in that orientation. This is not safe and is a violation of the Americans with Disabilities Act (ADA) regulations because you rock dangerously towards the front when the van comes to a sudden stop, even if you are restrained. Sudden acceleration creates a similar problem. The requirement that they send a bus rather than a van was in my profile, but they sent a van anyway sometimes. One day, the issue came to a head when one of the drivers refused to drive me because he knew he would be violating the ADA rules. That was resolved only by me accepting responsibility and explaining that my wife was extremely agitated and could not wait for another bus. Ensure that your Paratransit provider knows that you need a bus rather than a van if you use a scooter or large wheelchair.

When in a Paratransit bus, your mobility device is secured to tracks installed on the floor with ratcheting belt devices that fit in the tracks and connect to the scooter or wheelchair at four points. A picture of this method of securing my motorized scooter is shown on the top picture below using the Q'Straint system.* Other companies such as AMF-Bruns and Titan have similar systems.

It isn't obvious where the restraints should be connected to the scooter so

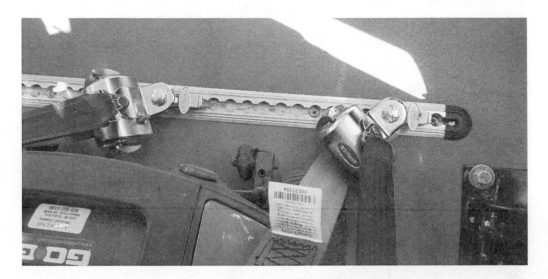

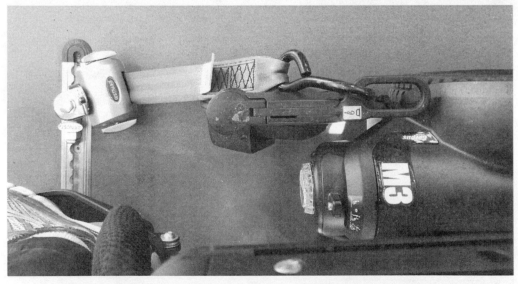

Top: **Paratransit Q'Straint securing system on motorized scooter.** *Bottom:* **Paratransit Q'Straint securing system on motorized wheelchair (photographs by the author).**

---

* View Q'Straint products at https://www.qstraint.com/.

different drivers do it in different ways. You should be aware of where to attach restraints to your scooter and tell the driver if necessary. Wheelchairs have obvious attachment locations as you can see in the bottom picture on the previous page.

Despite all the negatives, it is invaluable to have this transportation option for your needs on weekdays. Your local Paratransit system might be run more efficiently than mine so you might not experience some of these problems. Recently, a new contractor is operating our Paratransit system, resulting in improvements. Their plan to install a system where you can track your bus would solve many of the current issues. (That was not in place while we used Paratransit.)

The next section discusses the ultimate solution for vehicle mobility, handicap driving.

Learning to Drive with Handicaps

"Never, never, never give up."
—Winston Churchill

This section has six chapters. In the first, Chapter 20: Don't Assume You Can't, Most Can, I explain why I hadn't learned to drive earlier and the preliminary steps I took to develop a plan to learn how to drive again.

In the second, Chapter 21: Certified Driver Rehabilitation Specialist (CDRS®), I describe the best way to verify that you can drive, the type of testing a CDRS® does, and the hand control specifications they provide.

In the third, Chapter 22: Vehicle Modification and Selection, I offer suggestions and information to help you select the appropriate vehicle.

In the fourth, Chapter 23: Controls Installation CA: It Shouldn't Be This Hard!, I relate the lengthy, problem-filled challenges we faced to get the hand controls to work with the controls of the van I purchased.

In the fifth, Chapter 24: Controls Installation AZ: Will the Problems Never End?!, I reveal that after the problems were supposedly resolved, and we had moved from California to Arizona, some of the old problems returned and new ones appeared. This became a mystery story.

In the final chapter, Chapter 25: Training, DMV and Insurance, I convey information on the final steps to achieving the goal of driving again.

20

Don't Assume You Can't; Most Can

Great difficulties may be surmounted by patience and perseverance.
—Abigail Adams, in letter to husband John, November 27, 1775

As a reader of this book, you might have wondered why thirty months passed before I learned to drive with hand controls. The reason is that I just assumed, without doing adequate research, that with weak hands and no ability to use my legs, driving was impossible. In most other cases, I had thought ahead about what I was going to experience and did the research required to solve whatever problems might arise. Then I took action. That did not occur when it came to handicap driving.

Thinking ahead wasn't the problem. Sensing that my driving might end soon, I watched videos of people driving with hand controls even before I stopped driving. They used devices attached to the pedals to control acceleration and braking that worked with a push-pull action by the left arm. A steering wheel spinner controlled by the right arm was used for steering. I even bought some simple hand controls on Amazon, but several issues came to mind right away. What are the legal consequences in case of an accident? What are the insurance implications and notice responsibilities? What are the DMV requirements?

I decided to drive at low speed on my street and adjoining streets with these simple controls and seek answers to the questions later. I found that it was not easy to accelerate and brake smoothly, but I understood that those skills could be learned. However, with both hands occupied, it was impossible to use other control features usually controlled by one's hands, like turn signals and windshield wipers. How could I safely and legally drive with that restriction? Also, the drivers I watched on YouTube had good upper body strength. That was not the case for me.

At this point, I failed to do enough research. As explained earlier, my condition (Inclusion Body Myositis or IBM) greatly weakened my hands, wrists, legs and other muscles. My legs were useless for driving and with weak hands, there was a risk they would lose their grip. I also knew the hands were only going to get weaker over time. The inability to use turn signals, windshield wipers, blow the horn, switch between low and high beams, and turn on the windshield washer

120

combined with muscle weakness made it seem obvious that there was no way for me to drive safely.

Seventeen months passed before I got a lead that put me on the path to driving again. Throughout my journey, the support group I discussed earlier in this book has been immensely helpful. In this case, Joel Elmore, one of my golf group friends, put me in touch with his friend, who was driving with hand controls even though he has progressive weakness in all of his muscle groups. Like me, his hands are weak. One of his many helpful suggestions was to attend an Abilities Expo that was to occur in the San Francisco Bay area. It would be held in late October 2018, which was only a couple of weeks away.

My neighbor, Steve Steen, offered to drive us to the Abilities Expo, where he picked up pamphlets and other materials that would be useful later. At this expo, I learned about Certified Driver Rehabilitation Specialists (CDRS®) who can evaluate you and select the controls you need to drive safely. I was able to get the names and contact information for some of the local CDRS® agents.

I also learned more about motorized wheelchairs, including the pros and cons of the various drive wheel types and the control options available. I was able to test drive some of them. I met a representative from the company that would later sell me my wheelchair. I discussed with him what he recommended.

Also, I met the representative of the company that would install the controls in my van. I got his thoughts on the van that would be best for me and on the best wheelchair choice. His recommendation was different from what the wheelchair supplier recommended because he was more focused on maneuvering it in a van.

The recommendation to attend the expo was extremely helpful. Joel's friend helped in many other ways. He emphasized how important it was to get the elevation option for my wheelchair. He warned me against a front-wheel-drive wheelchair which I was considering. He recommended the Permobil M3, a mid-wheel drive wheelchair that I later purchased. He also told me that I would want a docking station instead of securing the wheelchair with straps. I would have come to the same conclusions on my own after more research, but getting that information at the beginning shortened the decision process.

I regret very much having done insufficient research early on. Jodie and I lost almost thirty months during which our life could have been much more fulfilling and with less dependence on others. This example applies to everything you might face. Don't just assume you can't do things. Resources and technology are available that might aid you in achieving whatever you hope to accomplish.

According to the Ability Center,[1]

> Joysticks have revolutionized the handicap driving experience for the severely disabled. Quadriplegics and individuals who can move no more than two extremities can now safely operate a handicap accessible vehicle.... Steering controls, gas and brake, turn signals, windows and doors, transmission selector and other accessible vehicle operating features can be tailored to your needs....

After doing adequate research, I learned that driving controls can handle many situations, including those more severe than mine. This was confirmed when I met a 4'2" below the knee amputee who has minimal hand function. Her fingers were webbed/fused when she was born. After multiple reconstructive surgeries, she now has four separated fingers on one hand and three on the other, but they are all deformed. As a result, she has significant problems with dexterity and getting a firm grip on objects. She can drive because she has good upper and lower body strength, is very agile, and has above the knee mobility. She can bear weight on her stumps. She drives a four-wheeled scooter into a Honda Odyssey minivan with an electric ramp, secures the scooter behind the driver's seat, and moves between the front seats into the driver's seat where she drives with hand controls.

This section of the book describes the process I followed to be able to drive with hand controls. It is viable if your mobility device is a wheelchair and you are without good upper body strength. However, because it is very expensive, you have to consider whether you have the means to afford it, and a strong belief that you will be able to drive for some time. Part of my rationale for incurring this expense was that I needed a van like the one described in this section to accommodate my wheelchair even if I couldn't drive, so much of the cost would be necessary anyway. You can save money with a smaller vehicle if that would work for you, or by buying a used vehicle that has already been modified.

If your medical condition is different from mine, there are other options outside this book's scope that you could consider. For example, I saw a man on YouTube who was strong enough to hoist himself out of a manual wheelchair into the driver's seat from outside the vehicle, then fold the wheelchair and put it in the back of his vehicle.[*]

Some innovative products might be helpful to you other than what I used. One example is a product called LINK[†] by Adapt Solutions[2] that can assist you in entering the driver's seat. Another of their products called Asento—XL-Seat[‡] can help you get into the driver's seat and place your wheelchair in the back.

One option I learned about while researching this book is Featherlite[§] hand controls by Sure Grip.[3] It relies on the fact that most vehicle manufacturers no longer use a throttle cable to link the gas pedal to the engine throttle. Instead, they use a computer-controlled throttle-by-wire system that uses an accelerator pedal position sensor. Featherlite takes the vehicle's throttle signal and connects it to the hand controls located on the steering column. A switch allows you to decide whether to use the hand or foot controls. Since no rods are connecting to the foot pedals, there is more legroom for the driver. Their push/rock system allows you to keep two hands on the steering wheel and be close to secondary controls like turn signals. If I had learned about Featherlite before I visited with the CDRS[®], I would have explored with the representative whether that would be a better option. It might not have changed the decisions she made because the floor-mounted controls put your hand closer to your body, allowing for greater

---

[*] In this and other cases where you enter the driver's seat from outside the car, you need steering column mounted controls; floor mounted controls would be in the way.

[†] See video https://adaptsolutions.com/product/link/.

[‡] See video at https://www.adaptsolutions.com/product/asento-xl-seat/.

[§] https://www.suregrip-handcontrols.com/featherlite.

leverage. However, one of the problems I have with my current controls is that secondary controls, e.g., turn signals, are not very satisfactory, as explained in subsequent chapters. The Featherlite system would have alleviated that problem.

I recommend that you do additional research beyond what I have provided. Attend an Abilities Expo and visit a company like Mobility Works to discuss the available options that would best fit your situation.

The next chapter provides information about what is involved and the value of a CDRS® evaluation.

21

Certified Driver
Rehabilitation Specialist (CDRS®)

*"Courage and perseverance have a magical talisman, before which
difficulties disappear and obstacles vanish into air."*
—John Quincy Adams, in speech at
Plymouth, Massachusetts, December 22, 1802

Certified Driver Rehabilitation Specialists evaluate your muscles' strength
and many other factors to determine the specific controls needed for you to drive
safely. There are a limited number of CDRS®s in the United States.[*] They are concentrated in urban areas, so you might have to travel some distance to get to
one. There are different levels and types of controls to use when driving. Some
examples include: Push/Rock, Push/Right Angle, Push/Pull, Push/Rotate, and
Electronically Assisted. Depending on your handicap, one type would be more
appropriate than the others. In my case, Push/Pull was better because of my limited finger dexterity and wrist weakness. More information is available on the
Ability Center website.[1]

Your local CDRS® might not have a vehicle equipped with the controls you
need or a vehicle large enough to conduct a driving test. That was the case for me.
At the time I was evaluated, I lived in the San Francisco Bay area. There were several CDRS® nearby, but none were capable of assessing me due to their vehicles'
size and the limited controls in them. I had to go to Sacramento, 80 miles away, to
get a CDRS® who had a fully equipped van with the control options needed. Neither my wife nor I could drive, so our son, Mike, flew up from Phoenix to take us.

The National Mobility Equipment Dealers Association (NMEDA) has pro-
duced a video[†] that summarizes the evaluation process. At the time of my test,
I had not seen the video referenced above[‡] so I was surprised by the extent of
these tests. I expected muscle strength evaluation but had no idea that I would
spend hours answering written and verbal questions. Nor did I expect to take
high-speed computer examinations that tested my cognition, reaction time,
peripheral vision, ability to avoid distraction, and many other factors. In one test,

---

[*] There are only 370 active CDRS® in the U.S. and Canada. Search for one in your area with this address:
https://www.aded.net/search/custom.asp?id=2046.
[†] https://www.youtube.com/watch?v=K8G2D4grpLs#action=share.
[‡] My test was even more extensive than the video suggests.

my reaction speed was measured by how quickly I could decide whether the picture that just flashed by had a symbol of a car or a truck and where it was positioned, e.g., at two o'clock, five o'clock, etc. Another test measured shades of color as they faded until I couldn't read the text. Based on these tests, the CDRS® created a preliminary specification for the controls, which was then checked and modified during the road test.

Due to my weak hands, the devices specified for me did not depend on hand or wrist strength but rather my more muscular arm and shoulder strength. An electronically assisted steering wheel was specified to minimize fatigue during driving and to plan for further strength deterioration over time. Acceleration and braking force were also electronically reduced for the same reason.* A control button on the driver's door was specified to activate turn signals and other functions. A left elbow bump against the button would initiate the readout of available control options, e.g., "right turn," "left turn." A second bump when the desired action is heard initiates the control.

The testing in the office was far more time-consuming than the driving portion of the test. After the bank of tests, I did some actual driving using hand controls. The road test was short, but as I drove, I gained confidence in adjusting to the acceleration and braking sensitivity. I was pleased that my CDRS® changed the hand controls from those she had intended to specify to another type after seeing what worked best for me.

My son made an insightful comment after the testing. Mike said that his concerns about me driving were alleviated by the rigorous examination administered by the CDRS®.

Once the controls are specified, vehicle selection is the next step. The company you choose for controls installation will be helpful in this decision. They usually have modified vehicles of different makes, and that experience will help in your decision process. The next chapter provides information on the factors to consider when choosing a van.

---

* As will be explained later, the modifications needed to reduce the force needed were expensive, increased the installation time and caused conflict with the van's control system that took a long time to resolve.

22

Vehicle Modification and Selection

Genius, that power which dazzles mortal eyes,/Is oft but perseverance in disguise.
—Henry Austin, the opening lines of "Perseverance Conquers All," in *The Business Philosopher* (March 1911)

Once you have received the specification for the controls from the CDRS®, there are three steps to follow when acquiring the modified vehicle best suited for your situation. The first is deciding which van to buy, including the make and model. Based on my size and the size of my wheelchair, the CDRS® thought the best options were the Toyota Sienna, the Dodge Caravan or the Chrysler Pacifica. Any of these three choices could accommodate a significant drop in the floor level. Conversions of Honda and Ford are also available.

The next step is to select a conversion. The vehicle has to be modified to make it wheelchair accessible. The floor is lowered, a ramp installed, methods for securing the wheelchair added, and the back seat area modified to allow for wheelchair maneuvering. Also, the means to enable the van to tilt toward the ramp when the ramp is deployed is installed.

The two largest companies that outfit wheelchair-accessible vehicles are BraunAbility and Vantage Mobility International (VMI). Modified vehicles are certified by the National Mobility Equipment Dealers Association's Manufacturer Quality Assurance Program and its safety-based Compliance Review Program. To get a comprehensive understanding of the extent of these modifications, watch a video of the VMI process on YouTube.[*]

How far the floor level is dropped depends on the vehicle chosen and whether you select a VMI or Braun conversion. All the Toyotas from Braun have a 14-inch dropped floor, and all the Toyotas and Chryslers from VMI have an industry-high 15-inch dropped floor designed for big and tall adults in large wheelchairs. Dodge conversions can have either 10- or 14-inch floor drops.

To determine which dropped floor would be best for you, measure how tall you are when seated in your wheelchair. If you are higher than 52 inches, you

---

[*] https://www.youtube.com/watch?v=gRhUVi0_0-k.

should have the floor lowered by 14 inches or more. If you are lower than 52 inches, a 10-inch dropped floor might be best to ensure good visibility.

The first two steps are best accomplished by working with a company that installs the controls because they usually keep an inventory of vehicles with various conversions. I decided to use Mobility Works to install my controls. One of the Mobility Works offices is located next door to Access Medical, who would be supplying my Permobil M3 wheelchair, so it was possible to check the various van and conversion options with the wheelchair I intended to buy. I arranged trials to determine which vehicle and modification would be best for me. For one trial, I invited the CDRS[*] who would do my driver training to attend to get his opinions and recommendations.

The third step is to decide whether you will drive from the wheelchair or the factory seat. Each requires different modifications. I will now explain what modifications are required to accommodate your choice. I will also discuss what's necessary for someone else to drive when you are a passenger. Finally, I will explain what changes are needed to alter your driving method from the factory seat to the wheelchair. That is more likely than switching from driving from the wheelchair to the factory seat.

Driving from the Wheelchair

To drive from the wheelchair, you first have to remove the driver's seat and the factory base on which it is mounted. Removing the driver's seat and its factory base takes only a few minutes. Unplug the power cable and pull up on a strap to roll them out as a unit, after which they can be taken down the ramp. In the video I mentioned earlier, you can see the seat removal process about 5 minutes and 45 seconds into the video. To secure the wheelchair, an EZ lock would be installed in the driver's seat area along with a stabilizer bracket in front of the EZ lock to keep the wheelchair from rocking back and forth.[†]

Another driver can drive the van as long as the seat and base are available. Putting the factory base and seat back in is easy. You reverse the process used to remove them. If you ever want to be a passenger in your wheelchair in the back, the wheelchair would have to be secured to securement strips on the floor, which are included with the van conversion. An AMF-Bruns system or equivalent would be used to secure the wheelchair and should be supplied when your van is delivered.[‡] A van seatbelt would secure you.

---

[*] The CDRS[*] who trained me was not the same one that tested me. To avoid the expense of having the one from Sacramento travel an hour and a half away at $100/hour, I used one who was more local.

[†] I wasn't told about the stabilizer bracket until after I bought the van and did more research for the book. Apparently, it is difficult to engage both the EZ lock and the stabilizer bracket at the same time. You must come in to them very straight.

[‡] You can't have EZ lock in the back to secure the wheelchair when your mode of driving is from the wheelchair because it would interfere with moving the wheelchair into a position to drive, thus the need for the Bruns system or equivalent when you are a passenger.

Driving from the Factory Seat

If you are going to drive from the factory seat, the seat must be removed from the factory base and installed on a 6-way base. The seat retains its limited ability to move up and down, forward and backward, and tilt the backrest. The 6-way base* has the extra capability to move the seat partially into the backseat area, rotate, and change elevation. An EZ lock would be located in the back so that the wheelchair can come up the ramp behind the passenger seat and, after engaging the EZ lock, rotate so that it is facing to the front-right. The 6-way base can then bring the driver's seat back and rotate the chair close to, and parallel with, the wheelchair. If your wheelchair has seat elevation as an option, the elevation of the factory seat and the wheelchair seat can be adjusted such that a slide board (aka a transfer board) can be placed between the wheelchair and the driver's seat with a slight downhill slope in the direction of the transfer.[†] If the wheelchair has no seat elevation, it is possible to perform the slide transfer using the 6-way base elevation. Depending on your strength, you may not need a downslope transfer.

Converting from Driving from the Factory Seat to the Wheelchair

If you start by driving from the factory seat, it is possible to make modifications to allow you to drive from the wheelchair at a later date. However, the 6-way seat base that is necessary for a slide transfer is not as easy to remove as the standard seat base. The EZ lock would have to be moved to the driver's seat area and a stabilizer bracket installed in front of the EZ lock. I'm hoping that I will never have to drive directly from the wheelchair, but I have demonstrated it is possible during the dry runs.

Van-Wheelchair Trial Results

There were multiple reasons for the van-wheelchair trials. I wanted to determine which vehicle would be best in two situations. For my primary use, I would drive from the factory seat and slide transfer from the back. Alternatively, for long trips, I could be a passenger and stay in the back in the wheelchair. The vans available for the trials didn't have 6-way seat bases[‡] so I couldn't perform slide transfers during the dry runs. However, during my CDRS® road test, I found that I could enter the van from the right side behind the front passenger seat with my scooter. The CDRS® van had a 6-way base and I found that it was easy to do a slide

---

* The name 6-way means it can move forward, back, up, down, rotate left, and rotate right.
† Pictures showing this process will be found in the next chapter,
‡ It is too expensive to put these in their inventory vehicles. They are added only when they get an order for one.

transfer into the driver's seat even though the scooter didn't have the helpful ability to change elevation as my wheelchair does. That alleviated any concern I had about using a slide transfer from the wheelchair.

I chose the slide transfer method because retaining the factory seat allows anyone to drive the van in the usual way on their own or with me in the back as a passenger. However, if I were unable to slide transfer because of my progressive disease, I wanted the ability to remove the front seat and drive from the wheelchair.

I tried the Toyota Sienna, the Chrysler Pacifica, and the Dodge Caravan. The VMI Chrysler Pacifica and the VMI Toyota Sienna both had adequate room in the van for maneuvering. There was less room in the Dodge. We learned that driving the wheelchair into the driver's seat with the factory seat removed was tight on the left. I couldn't quite center on the steering wheel. Some driver's door modifications would alleviate that problem if I later decided to drive from the wheelchair. It was unnecessary to make door modifications unless, and until, I had to drive from the wheelchair. Not making the modifications allowed better functionally while driving from the factory seat. In particular, the left armrest and some Toyota controls on the door could remain in place.

I selected a new 2019 Toyota Sienna XLE with VMI Northstar Accessible Conversion because the Chrysler conversion was still new and had been having recall issues, according to Mobility Works. I was able to drive a Permobil M3 wheelchair into the VMI modified Toyota Sienna with a 15" floor drop.

Pictured below is the van I purchased. The ramp is stored in a pocket under the floor of the van.

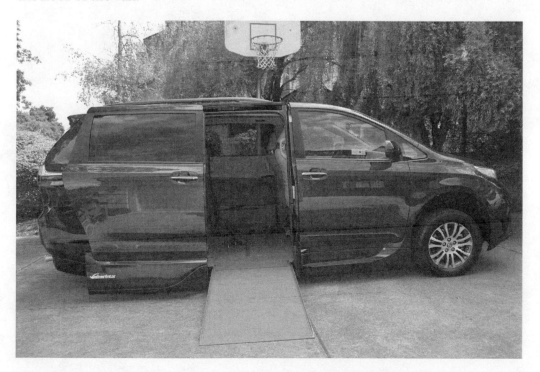

Toyota Sienna back-side entry (photograph by the author).

Right before I signed the contract, I learned that the modified van's allowable cargo carrying capacity is limited. Even on the part of the Mobility Works agent, there was some confusion, but it looked like I would exceed the capacity. The paperwork seemed to indicate the capacity was 190 pounds. I weigh about 210 pounds and my chair weighs 390 pounds. We later determined that the carrying capacity is 940 pounds, not 190 pounds. The 940-pound capacity isn't high either, but acceptable. This is something you will want to determine before you make your decision. If you have a smaller chair, the carrying capacity should be less of an issue.

The next step in the process is getting the controls installed and working properly. It took months to accomplish this, but it shouldn't have. That adventure is described in the next chapters.

23

Controls Installation CA

It Shouldn't Be This Hard!

"Just remember, you can do anything you set your mind to, but it takes action, perseverance, and facing your fears."
—Gillian Anderson, in the foreword *to Girl Boss:
Running the Show Like the Big Chicks* (1999)

Once the CDRS® specifies the hand controls, the company installing the controls acquires and installs them. Because my CDRS® specified a reduced effort steering system, the steering column had to be removed from the van and sent to Vantage Mobility International (VMI) for further modification. After that time-consuming process, Mobility Works conducted a "first fitting." The objective was to find the best locations for the controls with me in the driver's seat of my vehicle. They also had to find the best place for the EZ Lock to secure the wheelchair. When the wheelchair is engaged in the EZ lock, it has to be possible to rotate the wheelchair so that it is close to, and parallel with, the driver's seat when the driver's seat is brought back and turned to facilitate a slide transfer into the driver seat.

The picture on the right shows the EZ lock installation location determined by the "first fitting" and some of the securement strips that would be used with the AMF-Bruns system if they were needed. The picture on the following page shows the wheelchair about to engage the EZ Lock.

To utilize the EZ lock, a pin must be installed under the wheelchair to engage the EZ Lock. The pin creates a potential interference problem when the wheelchair goes over an abrupt

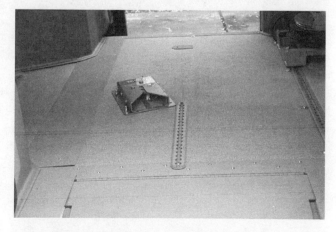

EZ Lock and securement strips (photograph by Marc Duquette).

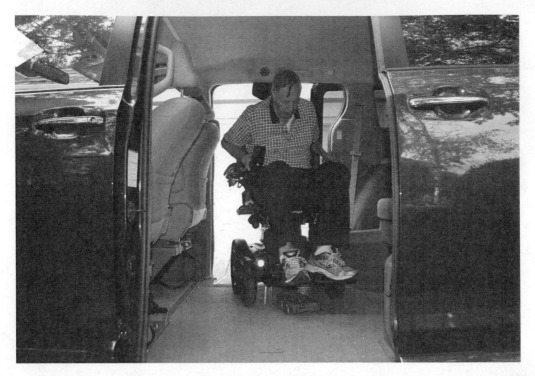

Engaging the EZ Lock (photograph by Marc Duquette).

elevation change, such as a threshold. After the EZ lock connection was installed in my wheelchair, I had a representative from Permobil, who sold the wheelchair, check the location of the pin as I went over a threshold into the house. He said it was going to hit, but because of the mid-wheel drive, the pin that would have interfered with the threshold was lifted by the wheels and did not impact the threshold.

The biggest test was when I got off a ramp from the Paratransit bus. The ramp came down at a downslope angle to an up-sloping driveway, forming a V shape. This is the kind of abrupt elevation change that can be a problem, but there was no interference between the pin and the driveway. Being able to handle this abrupt change was another factor that confirmed and validated my mid-wheel drive wheelchair choice.

I was somewhat concerned about how the slide transfer would work because I didn't want the slide board, a.k.a. transfer board, to slide off and fall between the seats. I bought a plastic transfer board from Amazon to try it. I chose plastic, thinking it would be easier to slide on it. Because I could change both the wheelchair's height and the driver's seat, I could create a downslope for the transfer. The combination of the plastic slide board and the downslope made for a smooth transfer. The difficulty was getting the slide board out from under me. The solution was to put most of my weight on my thighs, very little on my buttocks. I found that grabbing and turning the slide board was more effective than trying to slide the board out after the transfer.

The following picture shows the start of the transfer.

After the controls were installed, the van was brought to my home for a "final fitting" where I could use the controls to simulate driving to see whether further adjustments were necessary. We established that the location of the hand controls would work; no changes were required.

The picture below shows a completed transfer and the location of the hand controls.

The other concern I had was that to use turn signals and other controls, I had to use the left elbow bump device to set off a series of commands. The elbow bump control is a Crescent Voice-Scan, which is a multi-function switch box. The term "Voice Scan" is misleading. The "Voice" is a computerized verbal listing of commands that starts with the first elbow bump. When you hear the command you want, a second bump activates the command.

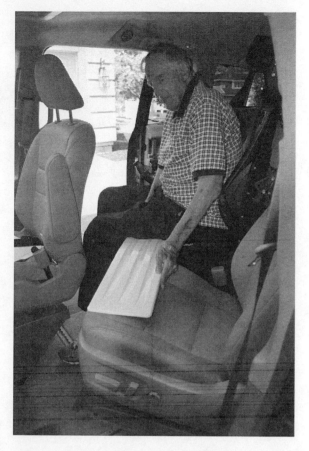

Start of slide board transfer (photograph by Marc Duquette).

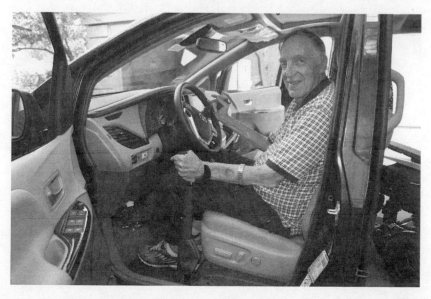

Driving position and hand controls locations (photograph by Marc Duquette).

The controls, listed in order, are right turn, left turn, horn, dimmer, cruise set, cruise on, wiper, and washer. I was concerned that this might not work because my arm position would change as I accelerated or braked. Thus, the elbow that would activate the control would also be changing position. Would I be able to use the voice scan at all arm positions? I was skeptical but was assured that the voice scan control was so sensitive that it would work. Furthermore, the CDRS® that specified the voice scan system seemed quite sure of her recommendation.

I had other worries about this system as well. Would I be able to respond quickly enough to choose the right command reliably? What would happen if I reacted too fast or too slowly and got the wrong response? What would happen if muddy water was thrown on the windshield and I had to go through multiple commands until I got to the windshield washer. I expected that it would take some time to use the voice scan system effectively, but I couldn't test it then.

As I mentioned earlier, one of the reasons I gave up on hand controls years earlier was the inability to activate windshield wipers and other controls because both hands were occupied with steering and operating the accelerator and the brake. The Crescent VoiceScan system solved some problems, but not others.

The obvious answer seemed to be voice-activated controls. For example, if you said, "Right turn," the order would be repeated. Once you confirmed it, the right turn signal would be activated. I was told that such a system existed but was prohibitively expensive, costing tens of thousands of dollars. One mitigating factor was that my vehicle supposedly had virtually all possible safety features. Blind Spot Monitoring (BSM) with Rear Cross-Traffic Alert (RCTA),[*] Lane Departure Alert (LDA) with Steering Assist (SA),[†] Pre-Collision System with Pedestrians Detection (PCS w/D),[‡] Dynamic Radar Cruise Control (DRCC),[§] Rain-Sensing Wipers (RSW),[¶] and Auto High Beams (AHB)[**] would minimize the shortcomings of the elbow control, and result in safer driving. In particular, RSW and AHB would avoid having to use the wiper and high beam controls. For long trips, DVCC would be valuable, but I don't expect to drive long distances. There is too much stress on the arms for that to be comfortable. As you will see, some of these features were in the van, some weren't, and some features were in the van but not working.

---

[*] The BSM uses rear bumper-mounted radar or ultrasonic sensors that detect other vehicles located to the driver's side and rear that are not easily seen with mirrors. RCTA shares the same sensors to check the right rear and left of the vehicle while backing up to prevent crashes.

[†] LDA uses forward-facing cameras to monitor the lane lines around the vehicle to alert the driver when the car approaches or crosses lane markings when your turn signals are not on. SA tries to keep the vehicle in the lane if it starts to exit the lane.

[‡] The PCS w/D system utilizes both radar and a camera to visualize and detect what is going on in front of the vehicle. It detects and alerts the driver to possible frontal collisions and when a pedestrian walks in front of the vehicle.

[§] The DRCC system uses a camera and radar to recognize vehicles directly in front of your vehicle and makes speed adjustments to maintain a safe following distance.

[¶] RSW work by installing a sensor on the inside of the windshield. It projects infrared light at an angle toward the windshield. The less light reflected back, the wetter the windshield. This information is used to turn on the wipers and to adjust their speed.

[**] Automatic high beam headlights use a photoelectric sensor to turn on and off the high beams depending on the light sensed from oncoming headlights, taillights and ambient light in cities.

The plan was to get the van in time to go to an annual family reunion in late June. This would allow me to take my wheelchair. But I learned that the van had to go to Toyota to integrate the van controls with the hand controls. Toyota's schedule wouldn't allow the van to be ready in time for the reunion, but it would be ready when we got back home the first week of July. I planned to start training at that time. However, when I got back, I learned that Toyota, VMI (who made the major van alterations), and Mobility Works (who added the hand controls) couldn't get the controls to work together.

As mentioned frequently in this book, it's not common for things to go smoothly. There was a significant delay in the delivery because those three companies were pointing fingers at each other.

It took a long time to uncover the real problem. When Mobility Works installed its electronics, they performed a lobotomy on the electronics of Toyota. This is not uncommon and is required. A contract between the VMI and Toyota requires Toyota to reset its controls once the van is modified and the hand controls are installed.* The local Toyota dealer ignored that contract and refused to make the changes based on the perceived liability if their controls did not function properly with a VMI modified van. I suggested strongly that there needed to be a conversation with Toyota USA to make sure that their franchisees honored the contract. Eventually, a different dealer agreed to solve the problem. I was told the problem was solved.

After waiting a month for the three companies to get the electronics to work together, the van was finally delivered in early August 2019. The timing was fortuitous because my brother Jim Reed and his wife Peggy arrived for a one-week visit the next day. This allowed us to check out the van and its controls. Jim could drive it the whole week, and I could get familiar with the vehicle and controls by test driving on local streets for a week. After a few minutes on the first drive, multiple warning signals flashed on, indicating that the electronics issues were *not* solved. "Pre-collision System Malfunction," "Check Brake System," "Anti-lock Brake System Malfunction," and "Lane Departure Alert Malfunction" were some of the warning signals. Most puzzling of all was, sometimes, no warning indicators appeared, then reappeared. The emergency brake warning light was sometimes on whether the brake was on or off.

When I saw that the elbow control was a round button, it was evident to me that it wouldn't always work. My elbow would be at different positions when I was applying the brake. A round button couldn't possibly be bumped in all of them, an obvious fatal flaw. I couldn't understand why any credible manufacturer could design something like this or why the CDRS® and Mobility Works thought it would work. As expected, it worked on level and uphill roadways but was out of reach on downhill roadways. My elbow was forward of the control button when I had to apply the brake, a predictable and unacceptable outcome. This device couldn't be round in shape and work effectively.

---

* Lowering the van affects the lane departure, blind spot monitoring, and other systems that were set to work at the normal height of the vehicle. The vehicle manufacturer must make the recalibration to ensure these systems work properly.

I drew up a design to add a rectangular device over the round control so it could be activated at any arm position. I reviewed the design with George Homolka, another friend with an engineering background. He made some improvements, and I submitted the design to Mobility Works. They were able to install a rectangular device that worked at all arm positions but of their design.

However, the system is far from ideal. You have to wait until you hear the action you want and acknowledge it with another elbow bump. That delay can be crucial. Furthermore, when you are concentrating on driving, it is easy to acknowledge too early or too late. The result is that you get an unintended outcome. For example, I sometimes got a left turn signal when I wanted the right turn signal. At that point, you confuse the drivers behind you, and you have to start over if there is time to correct the mistake. Occasionally, you bump the elbow control inadvertently, and you have to listen to the whole menu because you don't want to acknowledge any of the options. You can be distracted from your driving because of these issues, especially when driving with unfamiliar hand controls. I found this to be the most dangerous aspect of driving with hand controls. I had to train myself to ignore elbow control generated errors if I couldn't quickly correct them, but I got better at making corrections over time.

The instructions regarding how to engage the EZ lock on the wheelchair into the EZ lock mount were wrong and resulted in the wheelchair getting hung up on the EZ lock such that the wheelchair couldn't move but was not engaged. To assist my efforts to get the wheelchair to connect with the EZ lock, Marc, from Mobility Works, put blue tape on the floor to indicate the proper path. However, we still had difficulty getting the wheelchair to connect.

I was told that the solution was to increase speed and slam it in harder. It worked a few times, but eventually that created more problems than it solved. In one case, I ended up with the pin locked such that I couldn't move in any direction. Fortunately, Jim was there. With him partially lifting and me trying to drive out of the van, we solved the problem that time. However, it happened again, and we could not solve the problem without seeking immediate help from Mobility Works. It took quite a while, but we were instructed to locate a red, mechanical, emergency unlock for the EZ lock. That helped us get out of that situation. The technical staff advised me that we could potentially cause significant problems by coming in hard and fast; we should not do that anymore. They said that it should be possible to go in relatively slowly and still connect. Jim and I determined that the tape's line was not quite correct but found a path that worked much better.

Later I had Marc watch the process of the engagement, and he saw what the problem was. It seemed that you needed to have a guideline lined up in front of the EZ lock slot. We all thought that … wrong! It would have been true if the wheelchair could have entered in a straight line. But, it was necessary to make a slight turn to the left after entering the van. The pin moved enough out of line that the guideline wasn't accurate. That is why Jim and I had to find the ideal line by trial and error. I sent the van back so they could correct all the control problems.

We were told the mystery was solved after over two months of delays with incompatible electronics and multiple warning lights. The van was delivered again in mid–September. I insisted on getting an explanation that made sense to me. Since I have engineering training, I am not confident when told the problem is solved without a credible explanation, particularly when told a few times that it was fixed when it wasn't.

I had known that there were three companies involved, Toyota, VMI, and Mobility Works. But there were four companies. ColleBuilt provided the low-effort brake system, and all four companies had to work together to find the solution. The overview is that the reduced effort braking system didn't send a strong enough signal to be reliably read by the Toyota electronics. The result was that the Toyota electronics system sometimes detected a problem. A change Toyota made to their software about a year earlier when they put several warning indicators through one part of the software system instead of having different subsystems to catch various problems exacerbated the problem. The result was that multiple error signals were sent when only one "error" existed, making finding the problem more difficult.

The warning indicators resulted from a faulty reading from the brake actuator/force pedal switch, a Toyota part. The ColleBuilt low effort brake system did not consistently apply sufficient pressure on the Toyota brake force switch. When it didn't, it triggered the warning indicators in the Toyota system. ColleBuilt built a cable and turnbuckle retrofit kit to fit between the low effort brake system and the brake force switch. This allowed the technician to tighten the cable to apply the correct force on the brake pedal force switch. Too much and the warning lights go on, too little, and they also go on.

I was happy that we knew the cause of the problem. But, once again, I was concerned. The tension had to be perfect, and cables stretch. I assumed that it was only a matter of time before the tension would no longer be perfect. The good news is that if the warnings came back, I would know there is no real problem, and the cable tension could be adjusted.

But my optimism was unjustified. After thinking we had solved the mysteries of control installation in California, we moved to Arizona six weeks later. In the interim, I was focused on relocating and found little time to drive. Once in Arizona, I had a chance to use the van more extensively. The subject of the next chapter is the even greater problems and mysteries revealed there.

24

Controls Installation AZ
Will the Problems Never End?!

"Believe me, every problem has a solution. Some just take longer to figure out."

—Anonymous

The final van delivery occurred in September 2019, thirteen months after I went to the Abilities Expo and five months after the first demo. But the story doesn't end there!

It became obvious that my ability to care for Jodie, manage the household, and take care of myself was no longer tenable in our home. We decided to move to a senior living facility, but time was of the essence. The perfect apartment in the facility we chose was available, but we weren't the only ones interested in it. The short time frame to move and the complication of moving from a four-bedroom house to a relatively small two-bedroom apartment meant that I couldn't thoroughly test all the van features until weeks after we moved to Arizona in early November. When I finally focused on the van, I found out a few things.

1. The brake light started coming on again as it did after the first delivery, exactly what I feared would happen. I presumed the tension had changed and needed to be recalibrated.
2. The blind spot monitor wasn't working. I hadn't driven on freeways much previously and had assumed I just didn't know how to turn it on. That wasn't the case! It was on the window sticker list and the symbol was in the mirrors, but it wasn't functional.
3. The windshield wipers were not moisture sensitive as I had expected.
4. It appeared that the automatic high beam headlights were not working.

After realizing these issues, I worried about what else might not be working. I needed an expert to get to the bottom of all these problems to determine what went wrong, who was responsible, and how we could resolve them.

Since Mobility Works (MW) was responsible for the hand controls, I told them to find someone in Phoenix to resolve the problems. To their credit, they found Rudy to assist us. He is from AMS Vans, now a part of Vantage Mobility International (VMI), which modified the van as explained in Chapter 22. He was a great choice because Rudy is a real expert near us and because MW needs to maintain good relations with VMI. I could expect good cooperation. My son and I took the van to him for an initial examination.

   Rudy's assessment at that time is summarized below.

1. The cable approach for solving the conflict between Toyota's controls and Mobility Works' controls was not durable and caused the warning lights. A better solution was needed.
2. Some detective work would be required to find why the blind-spot monitoring (BSM) was not functional.
3. The van didn't have moisture-sensing windshield wipers. After examining the window sticker list, I realized that, contrary to my understanding, it didn't come with the van. I missed that somehow. Rudy told me that he could install an aftermarket device that would solve the problem.
4. Rudy recommended that we change the elbow control to eliminate all commands except right turn, left turn and horn. I readily agreed as I have never had to use anything except the turn signals and have frequently been distracted by the long list of controls actuated by mistake.

Before Rudy picked up the van for repairs, the windshield cracked. He recommended that the windshield be replaced first so that he could install the required sensors to the new windshield for the aftermarket rain-sensing system. There are also sensors associated with the lane-departure system on the windshield. Because Rudy had successfully worked with Safelite AutoGlass, I called them and was assured that they would be able to calibrate the lane departure sensors after replacing the glass.

When I brought the van to Safelite, they told me it would take an hour and a half to replace the windshield, so we went to a nearby restaurant for lunch. While we were eating, I got a call telling me that they couldn't calibrate the sensors because the car was modified (by VMI) such that it was lower to the ground than standard. They could replace the glass, but Toyota might not recalibrate the sensors because it wasn't factory glass. Rudy was surprised by their decision. He offered to pick up the van and have someone replace the windshield and calibrate the sensors while it was in his shop. He did so.

This whole investigation became an unbelievable mystery. It has been a long, frustrating experience to investigate and resolve all of these issues. As the investigation proceeded, the information and initial assumptions changed as new evidence came to light. In some cases, we don't know exactly what happened and might never know. Below I have summarized what we concluded and why for each issue.

Conflicts Between Toyota and MW Installed Controls

Once again, the ColleBuilt low effort brake system did not consistently apply sufficient pressure on the Toyota brake force switch, thus triggering warning indicators in the Toyota system. As I anticipated, the tension changed, but it was not the ColleBuilt cable and turnbuckle kit's fault. Instead, MW anchored the refit kit to a plastic part that flexed as might have been expected. The plastic flexing reduced the turnbuckle and cable retrofit kit's tension, thus lowering the force on the Toyota brake force switch. Rudy's solution was to anchor it to a stainless-steel plate and insert a gauge to determine the system's required force. This sounded rational to me. See the pictures below.

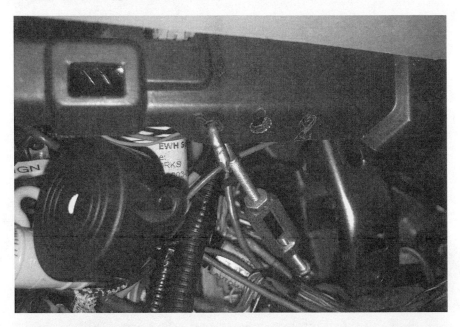

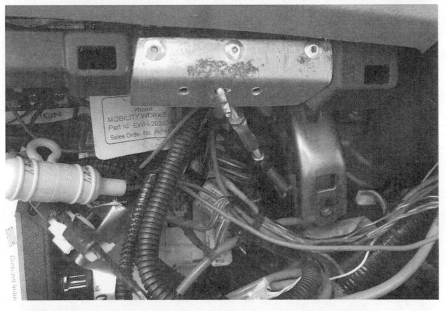

Top: Inadequate turnbuckle/cable connection. *Bottom:* Improved turnbuckle/cable connection (photographs by Rudy Quijada).

Blind Spot Monitor (BSM)

When Rudy picked up the van, he verified that the BSM was not working. Why not was a mystery for a long time because BSM was included with the van. Initially, Rudy saw some disconnected wires inside the dashboard and thought that BSM had been disconnected by VMI or Mobility Works. His initial conclusion was that Mobility Works removed the switch for the BSM and disconnected the wires. The switch was missing.

When he called Toyota to buy a replacement switch, they asked for the Vehicle Identification Number (VIN). Toyota told Rudy that my vehicle wasn't equipped with a BSM so they wouldn't sell him the switch. When told that the mirrors had the BSM symbol, Toyota suggested that someone replaced the mirrors or there was a factory mistake. Only after Rudy provided them with the equipment list and the window sticker did they agree to sell the switch. Rudy initially also thought the BSM sensors were missing from the back bumper.

Below are Rudy's conclusions regarding the BSM:

- The wires he thought were unconnected were not related to the BSM. They were associated with the Parking Assist system that was not part of the van package.
- We didn't need the switch he bought from Toyota. Switches were used in older versions of the Toyota van. The BSM is controlled differently in my van; it doesn't use a switch. Rudy put the switch into his firm's inventory.
- The sensors in the back bumper were not missing. One of Rudy's technicians thought they were missing because they looked different than he expected.
- Mobility Works knew the BSM system wasn't working. They contacted VMI, who told them to have Toyota fix it and send VMI the bill. VMI never received a bill for it and still had an open order for it. I have to assume that MW also has an open order for this item because it wasn't fixed.

The BSM system is working now, but why? Here is the reason. When VMI modifies a vehicle, electronics are disconnected. They have to be reconnected, and certain systems need to be recalibrated. The BSM system is one of them. The presumption is that VMI did not recalibrate the BSM. The fact that VMI took responsibility when MW notified them supports this conclusion.

Rudy disconnected the sensors and reconnected them. Then he had VMI recalibrate the BSM system. It works now!

What is still unknown:

- Why did Toyota initially say the van wasn't equipped with BSM?
- Why did Toyota sell the switch? They should have known it didn't need it.
- Why didn't MW get the BSM fixed and send the bill to VMI?
- Why didn't MW tell me that the BSM didn't work?
- Why did MW deliver the van to me in August 2019 without getting the BSM fixed?

Moisture Sensing Windshield Wipers

Rudy's investigation proved that there was no provision for moisture-sensing windshield wipers. While there is not much rain in Arizona for much of the year and most of my trips are short, I wanted to find a way to get this feature because I didn't want to have a sudden storm put me in danger.

Rudy said that he could solve the problem with an aftermarket device. After purchasing an aftermarket device, he told me that the system was rudimentary. It was based on the vibration that rain would cause. Usually, infrared light refraction is the means to detect moisture on the windshield. I was disappointed because a system based on vibration raised questions about whether it would sense misting or be inadvertently activated by road-induced vibration. He tried road testing it and found that it was not an acceptable solution.

Rudy found no aftermarket moisture-sensitive windshield wiper based on infrared technology. However, his connection with VMI, and theirs with Toyota, raised the possibility that Toyota would be willing to retrofit the van with their factory system. A retrofit would involve replacing the wiper control arm, installing the sensors and some wiring. Unfortunately, Toyota ultimately decided not to retrofit my van with its system.

After looking at several windshield wiper options for moisture sensing, we concluded that none of them were adequate. Rudy had been in conversation with Crescent Industries, who supplied the elbow bump system, and found an alternative to the elbow bump system. They use two sensors. The first step is to replace

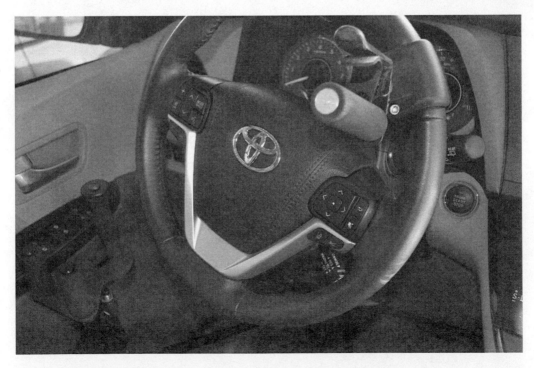

Tri-pin sensor system replacing elbow bump control (photograph by Rosemary Page).

the V-grip that had been placed on the end of the acceleration/braking control arm with a tri-pin mechanism that can be moved left or right on the shaft's end. The sensors can then be positioned so that a movement left activates one set of commands while a movement right activates another set. The picture on the opposite page shows the tri-pin installed in the lower left of the picture.

Initially, I was concerned about my weak wrists, which are among my body's weakest muscles. But movement left or right involves muscles other than the wrist.

This created new possibilities. I could eliminate some commands, e.g., cruise control, to avoid the long wait for the action desired, e.g., windshield wipers. I could choose whatever sequence of commands I wanted in each direction. By dividing the commands between left and right, an unintended initiation of the controls would start a very short list of possible actions.

I chose right turn, left turn, and horn for the left and windshield wipers and windshield washer for the right. The confirmation procedure for the left is another movement to the left when you hear the action you want. It is different for the right controls. If you acknowledge the windshield wiper with a movement to the right, the next two moves to the right increase wiper speed while the last one turns the wipers off. Acknowledging windshield washer turns it on. Holding to the right for a while when acknowledging it increases the amount of water sprayed on the windshield. Another right movement turns it off.

With this solution, I would be less likely to set off an unintended sequence of commands. Even if I did, the maximum number of possible actions I would have to listen to would be three. This would be much less distracting.

Although I do not often have to worry about sudden downpours where we live, I can deal with them by turning on the windshield wipers when necessary. This resolved all the outstanding concerns I had with the hand controls.

If I ever want to modify the system to add or delete controls, it will be easy to accomplish.

Automatic High Beams

Unfortunately, the automatic high beam headlight system has flaws that might make it useless for me. Since I can't use my hands to control the high beams, the idea that they could switch from high to low automatically was very desirable. After testing it, Rudy concluded that even low levels of ambient light turn off the high beams. He thought it might only be useful for long trips on highways. I will have to experiment with it.

Other Systems and Controls

Rudy tested all other systems and confirmed that they are all working. He also told me that I would only be financially responsible for the windshield replacement and the front-end alignment. He expects MW and VMI to pick up the balance.

Conclusion

Getting the hand controls installed was a time-consuming and frustrating experience. It is unlikely that you will run into as much difficulty as I did. For example, it is doubtful that there will be confusion concerning what features are included with the van but are not working; that screw-up was reserved for me! However, be sure that you get the features you need to drive safely in all situations.

Except for moisture sensing windshield wipers, I got all the necessary features, but that was a significant oversight. Fortunately, they aren't as critical to me because I live in AZ and don't drive very much. For much of the country, that would have been crucial. In any case, we found a good solution. Most of the controls you will want are on my van and are mentioned in this section for your reference.

The low effort braking and steering caused many of the significant problems. Depending on your condition, you may need low effort braking and steering, but if you do get them, expect difficulties unless a better solution has been found.

However, if they are specified and necessary, make sure you find a company that has done this successfully before. Companies like MW have many locations; make sure you go to one that has technicians who have done it before.

Here is another consideration. There could be two reasons why a low-effort system was specified. It could be that you need it now. But it could be that the reason it was specified is that it will extend the time that you can drive as your muscles weaken over time. In the latter case, think hard about the decision to have a low-effort system. Having one will delay getting a van ready to drive, cost more, and increase the chance of problems. If you are sure you will be driving for years and your strength will significantly decline, get the low effort system. Were I to have known what I know now, I would not have gotten the low-effort system.

I recommend that you avoid the elbow bump system. I have suggested some alternatives; others may be available when you are acquiring your vehicle.

The last steps in the process are training, dealing with the motor vehicle department, and insurance. These are covered in the next chapter.

25

Training, DMV and Insurance

"It always seems impossible until it's done."
—Nelson Mandela

Training for driving with hand controls turned out to be much quicker and easier than I expected. As mentioned in Chapter 23, the first delivery of the van was the beginning of August 2019, a day before my brother Jim arrived for a one-week visit. Jim knew I had an instructor brake on the passenger seat floor and was anxious to help me learn to drive with hand controls. I was able to practice driving with him every day for seven days. I drove only on local streets but learned how to accelerate and brake smoothly. While I couldn't use the elbow control for turn signals going downhill because it had not yet been modified, I could use it on level and uphill grades. I learned to ease up accelerating or braking while using the elbow control until it became second nature because a small mistake would be more easily correctable.* During that whole week, my brother never had to use the instructor brake.

We went out to lunch or dinner every day while Jim and Peggy were visiting. Jim did the driving for those trips because I wasn't ready to get out in heavier traffic. That much driving was an excellent test of the vehicle and immediately established the problems discussed in the previous chapters. While we had alarm signals of every kind it was clear that the van wasn't dangerous to drive.

Other benefits of having Jim drive were that it proved that another driver could easily drive the van the usual way. It also allowed me to get familiar with how to secure myself in the wheelchair when I was a passenger in the back.

Fortunately, I did not have to return the vehicle right away, which allowed me to take advantage of the opportunity for more training. After Jim left and before the van was returned, my neighbor Steve did some test driving with me, and I did some on my own. Before my CDRS® driver test, I decided to drive on some of the roads outside of my neighborhood so that when I was officially trained and tested, it wouldn't be the first time.

It wasn't until mid–September that the van was delivered with the modification intended to correct the control problems. That allowed me to schedule a

---

* By effectively coasting for a few seconds, I had time to think about what I needed to do with the control for braking or accelerating.

training session with Derrick Scott, the CDRS® I chose for training. Because of the training I had done with my brother, it took only one session before Derrick told me on September 17, 2019, that it was safe for me to drive. The following is his report.

> Mr. Reed completed 2 hours of behind the wheel instruction. During the session, Mr. Reed operated his own modified with adaptive controls vehicle. Driving conditions local residential, moderately dense commercial streets, and winding incline roads. Mr. Reed demonstrated adequate operational, tactical and strategic driving skills to continue independent operation of his vehicle.

There was some question about whether I would have to take a test at the California DMV when I started driving with hand controls. The CDRS® who tested me had said that you have to self-certify that you're changing from normal driving to hand control driving in California. She said she would provide me with a self-referral form for the DMV for reassessment. This is a proactive way of letting the DMV know you had a change in skills. She said that they may or may not test me but usually take her evaluation and training under consideration.

By the time I was cleared by Derrick to drive independently, we were already preparing to move to Arizona. When I asked Derrick what he recommended regarding the DMV, he said that since I was moving so soon to Arizona, it would be better to wait and get a driver's license in Arizona.

That worked out exceptionally well. After I moved to Arizona, all I had to do was fill out a form online with the Arizona Motor Vehicle Department (AMVD) for a Traveler's ID.[*] Then I went to AAA to register my Porsche Cayenne[†] and my Toyota and receive new license plates. While at AAA, I got the AMVD form notarized. The final step was to go to the AMVD where I got a driver's license with a Traveler's ID symbol on it that would not expire for five years ... without a written or driving test. While there, I got an ID with no expiration for Jodie. All this occurred in a couple of hours on December 6, 2019 ... some things are a lot easier in Arizona than in California.

As I started driving more in Arizona, I got better at not being distracted when using the elbow control for turn signals. Fortunately, I have not had to use any of the control options except "right turn" and "left turn" so far, and they are the first two control options in the sequence. (It was later the elbow bump system was replaced.)

There were no significant issues associated with insurance. I kept the insurance company updated on what controls were being installed, the modified van and hand controls' cost, and the date when the van was delivered. When we moved to Arizona, I supplied them with my Arizona driver's license number, the vehicle titles, and Arizona vehicle registration information.

---

[*] Arizona's Traveler's ID is the credential that complies with the federal REAL ID Act of 2005. The Travel ID will serve as valid identification to pass through airport security to board commercial aircraft as well as access restricted areas in federal facilities, nuclear power plants and military facilities. As of October 1, 2020, every adult needs to show a Real ID-compliant driver's license (or another acceptable form of identification such as a passport) to fly within the United States.

[†] I can't drive the Porsche but could be a passenger, if necessary, by using the scooter instead of the wheelchair.

While I still get a lot of help from my family, my ability to drive to my son's home, doctor's appointments, grocery stores, and drug stores ensures that I don't disrupt them as much with our care. When we go somewhere together, I can be a passenger while my son or daughter-in-law drives. Once at our destination, I am independent because I am in my wheelchair rather than my scooter, from which I would need assistance to get up. While the process of learning to drive with hand controls was time-consuming, frustrating, and costly, I am delighted that I did it. I am more independent and feel less of a burden to my son and his family.

(All of this changed with the arrival of Covid-19.)

The next section is about the challenges of being a caregiver. My wife, Jodie, has Alzheimer's. Providing adequate care for her overwhelmed me at times. I offer the solutions I tried that may be of value to you if you are a caregiver.

Caregiving from a Wheelchair

*"Caregiving leaves its mark on us. No matter what we do to prepare
ourselves the hole left behind looms large."*
—Dale L. Baker, in *More Than I Could Ever Know:
How I Survived Caregiving* (2014)

The preceding sections have primarily been about the effects of physical disabilities, the challenges they present, and their solutions. You would reasonably conclude that facing those problems were the dominant issues in my life, and you would be right. But the operative word is "were." Starting in July 2019, my priority shifted to caregiving for my wife, Jodie, who is living with Alzheimer's Disease.

Her caregiving presented the most significant challenges I had ever faced, and it overwhelmed me. I was distraught, depressed, and without answers at times. I broke down emotionally after a lifetime of being in full control. If you are a caregiver, you have likely experienced all of these emotions. That part of our journey started then, will continue while we are both alive, and will progressively become more difficult. Like every section of this book, I have provided resource information for those whose experiences differ from mine.

There are ten chapters in this section. The first, Caregiving Introduction, provides background information on Alzheimer's Disease and caregiving. The following chapters describe my experiences as a caregiver in our home in California and later at a senior care facility in Arizona.

26

Caregiving Introduction

"No disease should be allowed to have as its victims both the patient and the caregiver.
But that is exactly what is happening every minute of every day [with Alzheimer's]."

—Meryl Comer, in *Slow Dancing with a Stranger:*
Lost and Found in the Age of Alzheimer's (2014)

Alzheimer's Background Information

There are many excellent references concerning dementia and Alzheimer's Disease (AD). I suggest starting with two books. The first is a book by Jamie TenNapel Tyrone and Marwan Noel Sabbagh, M.D., called *Fighting for My Life: How to Thrive in the Shadow of Alzheimer's*.[1] All forms of dementia, including AD, take a massive toll on the patient and the caregiver. A wheelchair can solve an inability to walk because of a physical handicap. No such solutions now exist for AD. Both the patient and the caregiver suffer the anguish of witnessing the decline, knowing it is not currently possible to stop its advancement. However, there is some hope for the future.

In *Fighting for My Life*,[2] Jamie Tyrone describes her reaction when the results of a genetic test, taken for another reason, revealed that she had inherited two genes (APOEε4), one from each parent. She soon realized that meant she had a 91 percent risk of developing AD. Even though she had no symptoms of AD at that time, she experienced three months of depression at the prospect of getting that disease. Subsequently, she shifted from depression to a journey of discovery, participation in trials, and finally becoming an advocate for Alzheimer's research. She is an excellent example of the value of the approach this book recommends. After an adjustment period, while she was dealing with grief, Jamie accepted and adapted to her new reality. Commendably, she approached her challenges with a positive attitude and perseverance. As a result, she has made a significant contribution to AD research.

The other author, Dr. Marwan Sabbagh, is the Director of Cleveland Clinic Lou Ruvo Center for Brain Health in Las Vegas. He is a leading Alzheimer's and dementia expert and an investigator for Alzheimer's prevention and treatment trials. He explains that while there have been no recent breakthroughs for AD, "over the past ten years or so we've been making steady, incremental progress … we may be moving toward a model in which Alzheimer's may not be curable, but it is treatable."[3] He also reviews some of the promising drugs and trials that are underway.

Until there are breakthroughs, Dr. Sabbagh lists some things that can help delay the onset of AD. Some are well known and applicable to other health concerns. For example, a healthy diet, physical exercise, weight control, and a robust social life help those with heart disease and many other conditions as well as AD. Dr. Sabbagh also discusses the diets that can be helpful. To this list, Dr. Sabbagh added mental stimulation exercises. The discussion on mental stimulation exercises is informative because it is not what most would assume. Dr. Sabbagh indicates that trying new and challenging activities are more effective than crossword puzzles, for example. He provides a list of beneficial activities. It would be wise to research this subject if you are affected or believe you will be affected by AD.

The second book, *The 36-Hour Day, a Family Guide to Caring for People Who Have Alzheimer's Disease, Other Dementias, and Memory Loss*[4] by Nancy L. Mace and Peter V. Rabins, M.D., MPH, is in its sixth edition and has been a best seller. It is very comprehensive and an excellent resource for those caring for a person with dementia.

Another good source regarding the seriousness and extent of AD is the Alzheimer's Association®. Their website titled "Facts and Figures"[5] provides some "Quick Facts" and a link to their annual report.[6,*] I recommend that you download the full report from that page. There is a massive amount of useful information in this report, including helpful information on caregiving. A description of the stages of AD is included in their report.

You will find some insight into caregivers' challenges through helpguide.org.[7] Mayo Clinic also provides information on the various stages of Alzheimer's on a webpage titled "Alzheimer's Stages: How the Disease Progresses."[8]

According to the research I have done through these sources and others, I list some key information about AD below.

1. Alzheimer's is a large and growing disease, in part because we are living longer.
2. Over five million Americans live with Alzheimer's, and it is the sixth leading cause of death.
3. For seniors, its impact is even more significant. One-third of seniors die from it.
4. It kills more than breast cancer and prostate cancer combined.
5. While deaths from heart disease are decreasing, deaths from Alzheimer's are rapidly growing.
6. It impacts women and African Americans disproportionately.

---

* My reference to this report might be out of date because the report is issued yearly. Use the link to the Quick Facts website to find the link to the latest report in that case.

The Alzheimer's Association®, Mayo Clinic, and other sources describe the stages of AD. However, there are differences in how they define them. I recommend that you review these sources for details. As a brief overview, the mild stage doesn't significantly affect personal relationships or the ability to work. The memory of recent conversations and events is impaired, and sound decisions are difficult.

In the moderate stage, there is more confusion and forgetfulness. Knowledge of the day of the week is lost, and help with daily activities is required. Recognition of family members is impaired. Wandering becomes problematic. Behavior and personality begin to change.

In the severe stage, the ability to communicate coherently is lost. Daily assistance with personal care is required for bathroom issues, eating, and dressing. Eventually, physical abilities decline and can progress to an inability to swallow and incontinence regarding bladder and bowel functions.

My assessment of the status of Jodie in early July 2019 was that she was in the moderate stage of Alzheimer's dementia but also exhibiting the severe stage regarding the ability to communicate coherently.

Caregiving Background

I have listed some key information about caregiving below as gleaned from personal experience, the references mentioned in this chapter, and other sources:

1. There are about 16 million Alzheimer's caregivers in the U.S.
2. Family members and friends provide over 80 percent of senior caregiving in the U.S.
3. Caregivers sometimes experience grief more severely than the patient. They also suffer emotional, financial, and physical difficulties much more often.
4. Many AD caregivers experience depression, stress, anxiety, loneliness, and exhaustion.
5. Caregiving can overwhelm you.
6. Your patient's behavior and personality may change. Violent behavior is also possible.

Though there are millions of caregivers, we don't share the same experiences. Each situation is unique. Different patients exhibit different symptoms and personalities. In the next chapter, my description of a "non-compliant" patient will make this point clear. Many of the caregiving approaches suggested by the sources I have provided were not viable in my case because of non-compliance. Non-compliance was the most challenging aspect of caregiving for me. Yet, I didn't find much attention given to that subject. I'm sure there is a certain amount of non-compliance in most cases, but the extent of it varies widely. A caregiving relative of ours has virtually none. Nevertheless, the challenges she does face are also having a significant impact on her.

People love my wife because of her pleasant, humble, and caring personality. She compliments everyone. With AD, she has become non-compliant regarding many critically essential matters, including health and personal care—more on this in the next chapter.

Among the reasons that you might have become a caregiver for a relative or close friend are dementia, Parkinson's, blindness, a progressively debilitating disease, or physical limitations caused by an accident or surgical mistake. An Internet search will reveal abundant information on being a caregiver. There are common themes of great importance in any caregiving situation. Among them are:

1. Build a support team.
2. Prepare for emergencies.
3. Seek advice.
4. Ensure medications are taken on a schedule.
5. Take care of yourself.
6. Organize and simplify life.
7. Make your home safe.

One of my fraternity brothers, Dick Hamme, lost his wife in 2019 after a 13-year deterioration with Alzheimer's. Most of the time, he cared for her in their home but had to put her in a facility near the end. He told me, "Being a caregiver is exhausting, physically, mentally and emotionally. You can't do it alone. You need to involve a team to assist you and the patient. As the disease progressed I had an absolutely superlative support network: family, a support group, friends and neighbors, a church community, a daycare, the home where she lived, Hospice and a medical practice that truly understood the disease. All of these were essential in caring for Nancy, and caring for me."

My experience suggests that all of these items are important but none are as important as ensuring that the patient feels loved and is in what they perceive as a safe, comfortable environment.

As this book's content conveys, it takes a positive attitude (as difficult as that is at times), perseverance, and ingenuity to overcome the many problems you need to solve. When it comes to caregiving, you need all those attributes, but love is the most important. Love is what keeps you going. You want to help. You want to make them happy. You want to make them feel safe. Most of all, you want them to feel loved. That is the key not only for their satisfaction and behavior but for your success as a caregiver. The love comes back to you and helps you maintain your health, happiness, and sanity.

An AD caregiver watching a loved one morph from what was once a capable, intelligent, wonderful person into someone entirely different generates many intense, unfamiliar emotions. Our son, Mike, once told me that he had to think of his mother as a different person to deal with the changes in her and find new ways to communicate with her.

My own struggles in this regard hit home with great impact by an attachment to an email, as you will see by reading the paragraphs below.

In late April 2020, I opened my computer to see an email from Nancy Reed, my sister-in-law. She and my brother, Frank Reed, reviewed my book as I was writing it. Like the rest of our family, they were fully aware of the difficulties we had been having. Nancy is a gifted writer, whom I hope will publish her work someday. She said that she couldn't sleep the previous night until her feelings about our situation were expressed. The email included an attachment titled "Don't Leave—An Ode to a Caregiver." I started crying halfway through it and couldn't stop for about 10 minutes.

With her permission, I have included it below. Many caregivers will identify with this Ode.

Don't Leave—An Ode to a Caregiver
by Nancy Reed

Don't leave
Hold my hand
I recognize you
But I don't know your name
I see your tears
I want to comfort you
But I don't remember how
You work so hard
I want to help
But my mind gets all jumbled when I try
The music you are playing is beautiful
I can sing all the words
I see a small girl on a swing
She sings with me
I'd like to tell you about her
But I am so tired
She keeps fading away
When she comes back, I will
Don't leave

The impact on me was intense for so many reasons. I was greatly affected by how well Nancy captured how it feels to have the love of your life for over 50 years slowly slipping away. Jodie is sensing it too. She often asks if I am going to always be with her ... *"don't leave."*

Beyond that, it passionately describes the confusion Jodie must be feeling, the frustrating inability to express herself, and the vague knowledge of what is coming. Nancy knows how kind, caring and loving Jodie is and captured the concerns Jodie must have about my struggles and her inability to help me despite the desire to do so. Only someone who cares deeply about both of us, has great insight, and superior writing skills would be able to create an ode that says so much in so few words.

The next chapter discusses my caregiving experience while caring for Jodie in our home in California before her condition changed dramatically.

27

Caregiving at Home

Before the Crisis

"Love is, above all, the gift of oneself."
—Jean Anouilh, in *Ardèle* (1949)

This was a difficult chapter for me to write because it is about my wife, Jodie, whom I love very much. She won't read the book, but family and friends' reaction about a frank discussion of her situation and the effects on both of us concerns me. I had to put those concerns aside because the purpose of this book is to help others. If I am not candid, there would be little reason to include this section in the book.

First Signs, Testing, Changes in Cognition and Behavior

Jodie and I both noticed 15 or 20 years ago that her memory was degrading, albeit slowly. In 2007, she was referred by a neurologist to a psychologist to evaluate her. After she was tested, the psychologist concluded that she had a normal memory for someone her age. After we left the psychologist's office, we started laughing because we knew we had just wasted our time. It wasn't true! Jodie had been on a long-term, slow, but steady decline.

We went through the same process again in 2012. A different neurologist referred her to a different psychologist. Brain MRIs and MRAs were essentially normal.* The neurologist gave Jodie a choice of medications, but she would not take any of them due to her fear of medicine and distrust of doctors.

We went back to the same neurologist again in June 2016. This time the neurologist conducted the written and verbal testing herself instead of referring us to a psychologist. A series of tests covered a broad span of cognitive domains, including memory, attention, language, and visuospatial. Again, the brain was scanned. The scans revealed little change compared to the scans from 2012. Other than telling us that there was no tumor, we learned nothing useful.

---

* An MRI and an MRA are essentially the same test. Powerful magnets, radio waves and a computer are used to create two-dimensional or three-dimensional images of the inside of the body. An MRA is used to examine blood vessels while an MRI is performed to examine other parts of the body

Once I retired, I started taking on more and more responsibilities for household duties. By 2018, I performed all household duties, including providing meals. While we both have significant progressive diseases, fortunately, they are not the same. For some time, we had been able to help each other. Jodie always asked what she could do for me even when I didn't ask for help. Given my physical limitations, I often need help but what she could do to provide that diminished over time until there was almost nothing left. Eventually, I learned that asking for her help was counterproductive. To help you understand this, I will give an example that demonstrates the extent of her memory loss and disposition change.

It is time-consuming to close down my computer, get up from my lift chair, transfer to a mobility device, and use the lift to retrieve items from the refrigerator or elsewhere. Then I have to reverse the process. Also, when I am in a wheelchair, it is difficult to transport things because, unlike a scooter with a floor and one or two baskets, there is no storage capacity in a wheelchair. If Jodie were nearby, I might ask her to get a can of Coke out of the refrigerator. For a while, she was able to do this, but by the time I started writing this book, that was no longer true. She would want to help but might bring a book and some silverware instead of a Coke.

To deal with this, I tried giving her step-by-step instructions, e.g., "Go to the kitchen." Once she was there, I would say: "Open the refrigerator door." Then, "Get a can of Coke." As she regressed, that technique would fail at some point. I tried being more descriptive, e.g., "The Coke is in the black and red carton on the left side of the second shelf." It got to the point where she asked: "What is the refrigerator?" When I said it was the big silver thing in front of her, she would look everywhere but at the refrigerator.

I had not read the HelpGuide article or the other references in this section until after we left our home and moved into a senior care facility. I had developed the methods I used to manage Jodie's care through logic and a deep understanding of my wife through 53 years of marriage. In many cases, recommendations in the references were similar to my own, but not always. I will note the similarities and differences in this section.

Under Communication Do's, the HelpGuide recommends, "Keep communication short, simple, and clear. Give one direction or ask one question at a time" and "Speak slowly."[1] The Mayo Clinic[2] (Mayo) and the National Institute of Health's National Institute on Aging[3] (NIA) are other good sources of information, and they offer similar advice. The Mayo Clinic states: "People with dementia best understand clear, one-step communication."[4] NIA offers the same advice. "Offer simple, step-by-step instructions."[5] This is what I did and still do. Step by step, simple directions worked well for a while but then lost their effectiveness. I still try limited instructions in much simpler situations, but they usually don't work. Trying frustrates me and upsets her. Speaking slowly remains a useful strategy.

It quickly became obvious that the result of asking for help was very negative. It was nearly impossible to cover my frustration, much as I tried. If my words or expression showed my frustration, Jodie would pick up on that, get very mad and react negatively in various ways. In a review of the resources I reviewed, I found that they caution caregivers to avoid getting frustrated because the other person responds to body language and the tone of your voice more than what you are saying. This is excellent advice but difficult to always achieve.

I soon learned not to ask for help, but she still offers frequently. Usually, I tell her I don't need anything and thank her for her willingness to help. At other times, I let her do things because it allows her to believe she is helpful, realizing that this makes extra work for me. Mayo confirmed for me that this was a good approach by recommending: "Allow the person with dementia to do as much as possible with the least amount of assistance."[6] Unfortunately, I have to undo almost everything she does, e.g., take the dirty dishes back out of the cabinets where we store clean dishes. Despite this negative, I believe it is an important factor in keeping her sense of usefulness and well-being. Many times a day, I see her doing something that should not be done and will require me to correct. Sometimes I have to tell her not to do it, but avoid doing so when I can.

I think there were several reasons for her negative reactions. She thought I was indicating she was stupid; she wanted to help but was frustrated that she was unable to do so; or I was not appreciative of her attempt to help me. She was also in denial of her dementia and didn't want to accept that she had diminished capability.

There was another cause for very negative reactions. It wasn't just that she couldn't remember things. She started "remembering" things that never happened or was positive that she had never known things that she had been told many times. That was problematic enough, but she would get furious if I didn't agree with her.

The reactions to her sensing my frustration were reasonably mild. They could be verbal, or she might stomp out of the room and stay in the back of the house for a while. The reactions when I did not agree with her "memories" or told her that she had been told something she "never knew" were more significant. She was 100 percent sure she was right and was upset that I was "lying" to her. The reactions were always verbal and involved her making a tortured face and putting the fingers of one of her hands in her mouth and pretending to bite them. At times she would also throw things, sometimes at me. Occasionally, she would hit me or swing something that would hit me. Sometimes she would grab my arms and squeeze so hard they would bruise. Most of the time, I was in my lift chair and unable to get away from her.

I don't want to minimize the issue of violence, but it is important to put it into perspective. These incidents were brief periods during the day and didn't happen every day. Most of the day, every day, we were extremely happy. Many times a day, we told each other that we loved each other. Usually, the violent behavior was not very dangerous, but the risk of her unintentionally causing significant harm was present when she was out of control.

I tried to prevent physical violence by telling her that if she hit me, I would hit her back harder. For some time, this threat was effective, but it didn't last. The worst case was when she swung her purse at me. There was a metal chain on it, and it hit the bone surrounding my right eye. I escaped with some bleeding and bruising, but it could have been dire. My son worried about my safety.

I realized that if I couldn't control the violence, I would not be able to care for her. This would destroy us both. I had to do something to stop the violent behavior so I could safely continue to function as her caregiver. After she damaged the region near my eye, I decided to take drastic action. As soon as I could, I slapped her leg with an open hand so it would sting but not harm her. I made sure she understood why and told her that she was not allowed to hurt me. If she did, I would do it again. After a few more incidents, the violence stopped.

I don't think you will find this advice in any references. I expected some readers would strongly disapprove of my solution to this problem. So I wasn't surprised when some reviewers told me not to include this information. They understood that I would never harm Jodie and knew of the terrible consequences for both Jodie and me if I was so seriously injured that I could no longer be her caregiver. But they feared that some people would react in various ways, including legally. They had a valid point. During my research, I read *What to Do Between the Tears.... A Practical Guide to Dealing with a Dementia or Alzheimer's Diagnosis in the Family*[7] by Tara Reed. In addition to writing the book, she shared her journey on social media. A sampling of what happened to her is provided below:

> I once had someone tell me it was shameful that I would show a photo of my father in a "state of decline." She said she would be ashamed if her daughters ever did the same.... I questioned whether I had truly done anything disrespectful in regard to my father. I also cried....[8]

I did not research her social media account, but I am confident that my descriptions of Jodie's condition and my solutions are more candid than Tara's. I decided not to take my reviewers' advice. I strongly believe the best way to help those reading my book is to be candid about the problems I faced and how I dealt with them, even if that results in criticism. I mentioned my reviewer's caution to our son, and he said: "You probably will get blowback on this, but I completely agree with your decision to include this information."

But another reviewer's comment concerned me more. In effect, she said that some readers might not understand that I never have hurt Jodie and never would. Her concern was that some would believe that I was advocating violence to control behavior and would use it in abusive ways. So to be clear, *I do not advocate violence as a caregiving technique. I did not "hurt" her and never would have.*

I could have listed additional violent incidents. Instead, I revealed only enough to allow the reader to understand its significance. I knew that if I couldn't stop it, I couldn't care for her. I knew no one could do as good a job as I was doing. I knew that I would be devastated if I couldn't be with her and had to break my "for better or worse" vow. I knew the most important thing was the devastation and emotional harm that Jodie would experience if I weren't her caregiver. I don't believe it is possible to have a stronger, more loving bond than we have had for over 50 years. The betrayal she would feel would be indescribable. I don't think I could have stood seeing it in her eyes.

I hope you never have to face a choice like this, but you will not always find advice for the situations you are dealing with and will have to make your own decisions. My solution was effective, did not harm my wife or our relationship, and allowed me to continue as her caregiver to mutual benefit. One of the reasons you won't have to make the choice I did is because medication might have solved the problem, but Jodie wouldn't take medication due to the non-compliance issue discussed in more detail below.

It wasn't just memory and disposition that changed. She was non-compliant concerning medical issues and my attempts to help her. Paranoia, bathroom issues, and dressing became problems too. There were other challenges as well.

Non-Compliance

Like most caregivers, the challenges of caregiving have, at times, overwhelmed me. There were multiple reasons; however, the primary reason was that Jodie is a non-compliant patient. This is, by far, the most difficult obstacle to effectively caring for her. Some people are compliant in responding to help; others are not. I can't stress too much the importance of compliance. It is much easier to care for those who will respond positively to you because they will take medicine, get medical testing done, and follow instructions. Non-compliance affects everything.

Most importantly, it affects the ability of the caregiver to care for the patient properly. It dramatically increases the stress that both the patient and the caregiver experience when the caregiver attempts to provide effective care. The stress on both individuals can affect their health. If your patient is non-compliant like mine, you will be at more risk and need to find ways to reduce your stress.

While I was writing this chapter, I met a lady who was the caregiver for her mother until she died from Alzheimer's. She described that year-long experience as one of the best years of her life. She told me that her mother was very compliant and would do whatever she was asked to do. In my research, I had learned that some people find the experience of caregiving very gratifying. That same lady is now caring for her brother, suffering from amyotrophic lateral sclerosis (ALS), a.k.a. Lou Gehrig's disease. In the brief time I talked with her, it was evident that she approached these challenges with a great attitude, a continual theme of this book.

Unfortunately for both Jodie and me, Jodie is very non-compliant. She is suspicious of doctors and won't take medicine, blood tests, urine tests, bone scans, etc., so they really can't help her. Most of the time, she will not do what I ask when I am trying to help her and will react negatively to my attempts to help. I often wonder whether attempting to help is worth it when the result is a negative mood or behavior and the goal is unachieved.

She won't cut her toenails or fingernails and won't let me do it ... it's too scary! Once that led to an emergency room visit caused by the nails getting jammed back unto the flesh and causing a cut that got infected. The nails are so long her shoes don't fit and hurt her. When I took her to a podiatrist, she screamed, and it took three of us to get them cut. She wouldn't go again after that. Eventually, the toenails were forced to turn almost 90 degrees due to the pressure of the toenails against the front of her shoes. The picture below shows how bad the situation is.

This will result in a serious problem at some point, but no one can do anything about it now, although many have tried. She stopped taking showers and washing her hair over two years ago. My sister, Ellen Reed, was able to get her to a hairdresser once. Jodie's friend, Terry Totten, did twice, but it was very stressful. The second, and last time, was a disaster. It was never going to happen again. Terry didn't share all the details, but I know Jodie wouldn't sit while her hair was washed. The hairdresser had to wash Jodie's hair while she was standing up. The only reason even that was accomplished was that the hairdresser was Terry's friend; no one else would have been willing to deal with it.

Paranoia

Jodie always had a little paranoia. It got much worse when she declined mentally. She started to think the people on TV could see and hear her, so she whispers or hides in another room when she is concerned. She gives me trouble if I am not fully dressed, especially if there are women on the TV screen. In her mind, these people come out of the TV and do bad things in the house. She claims to have seen them, but when I ask her to show them to me, they have left.

Because she thinks terrible people come into the house, she hides things, often items critically essential to me. She is too good at this! We have found unexpected things in unusual places. One example is a pizza found under a sofa. There are some places I can't search because of my handicaps. For example, two of her favorite hiding places are under her bed and under the love seats in the living room. I can't get down to look under beds and have no access to the living room.

I have had friends, neighbors, family, and my handyman conduct searches for critical items many times. Immediately after she hides these things, she forgets

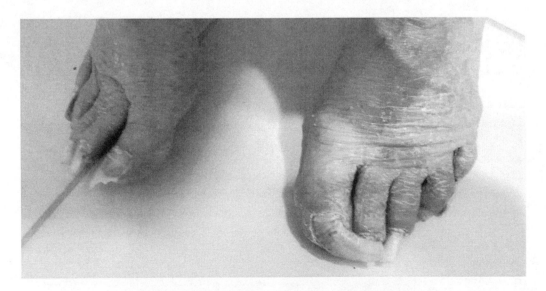

Distorted toenails (photograph by the author).

where she put them and even that she hid them. She always worries about what the trash collectors are doing and goes out sometimes to tell them to stop. I had to alert the company about the problem and advise them to ignore her comments. She also worries about what the gardeners are doing.

She is very anxious when people are in the house, especially those who go into the back. Our handyman and contractor are the best examples. At times she has been very unkind to them, which is utterly foreign to her usual disposition. Until we got the cleaning lady mentioned in Chapter 5, she thought the cleaning ladies were stealing.*

BATHROOM ISSUES

Bathroom issues became a serious problem as well. She started urinating in her clothing at night, sometimes on the rug in her bedroom and other times on the bathroom floor. When I heard noises indicating that she was having trouble, I got up and told her everything was okay; I would take care of her. I would give her clean and dry clothes. Then I would throw her wet clothes in the washing machine to be washed in the morning. Finally, I would sop up the bedroom rug as well as I could or dry the bathroom floor. Cleaning up while in a wheelchair is quite challenging. She also started urinating in wastebaskets. A couple of times, she even defecated in wastebaskets. That made the cleanup easier but was more disturbing.

To resolve this problem, I bought her incontinence underwear and hid her regular underwear. Getting her to wear them was a sometimes thing. When I was successful, they avoided the need for cleanup or made it a minor effort. The downside was that once she put them on, she wouldn't take them off. Small and medium leaks would be absorbed. After that, they were ineffective if she didn't change them. They are designed for one-day use.

After a few days, they would break and hang out behind her like a tail. She wouldn't take them off or let me do it. Even our daughter, Kris, couldn't get it done. At first, I gave her new ones assuming she would take the others off first. I was mistaken. She put the new ones on, but the tail of the old ones remained. I couldn't let her go out in public like that! The only solution was to trap her with my wheelchair in a corner, grab the tail and either cut it or pull hard enough that it would tear off. She resisted this by hitting me but not enough to hurt me. Simultaneously, she would call me the worst person in the world and other invectives. Ten minutes later, she would tell me how lucky she was to have me and how much she loved me, having no apparent memory of the event. I knew this would happen because of her short-term memory and over 50 years of a happy, loving marriage.

Another unexpected bathroom issue had to do with how she cleaned up after going to the bathroom. She has put concentrated laundry detergent, Windex, and other things on her private parts. They burned her. I hide these materials, but

---

* The Alzheimer's Association mentions that accusing people of stealing is typical for Alzheimer's patients.

somehow she finds them. Kris and I both bought some products that would not be harmful, but she didn't use them.

For reasons unknown, Jodie takes all the toilet paper out of the bathroom many times a day. It ends up in or on her bed, on nightstands and dressers, inside drawers, in the family room on end tables, and elsewhere. I have to check a couple of times a day to resupply it. When in the wheelchair, I can't get into the bathrooms she uses, which complicates things.

DRESSING

Getting her dressed to go to Renew (her religious group), an appointment, or lunch became time-consuming and contentious. Sometimes she wanted to put a blouse on her legs instead of pants. Sometimes, she put her bra outside her blouse. At other times, she put her underpants outside of her slacks. Because she hides things, I usually had to hunt for shoes to get her dressed. I dealt with this by hiding some of her clothing myself so I could get what she needed quickly and by getting her up hours early. It is stressful until I get her out of the door. Mayo Clinic recommends: "Anticipate that tasks may take longer than they used to and schedule more time for them."[9] Knowing this is the case, I still misjudge the time it is going to take to get her ready for many things.

OTHER CHALLENGES

In 2018, Jodie wanted to call her mother, who she suddenly believed still lived in Leominster, Massachusetts, her home while in high school. She asked for her number. She had to learn and relearn over and over that her mother had died in the '70s. She was very depressed during this period until she finally accepted it. That lasted for a while, but now she thinks her mother is alive again. If I can, I avoid correcting her to prevent her from getting depressed. The same issue arose after her brother (her last sibling) died. When she asks me whether Tom is coming, I just tell her no without further elaboration to avoid getting her depressed or have her challenge me on this point. Here is what HelpGuide has to say on this subject. "Use distraction or fib if telling the whole truth will upset the person with dementia. For example, to answer the question, 'Where is my mother?' it may be better to say, 'She's not here right now' instead of 'She died 20 years ago.'"[10]

I have to work hard to get her to eat sufficient amounts of nutritious food because she no longer likes things she used to enjoy. She can forget several times in one night what food has been prepared for her. Too often, she ends up eating a peanut butter sandwich and wasting what I prepared.

I don't want her to use the stove. We had a couple of close calls with her leaving the stove on with a pan on the burner. As explained earlier, it is not possible for me to quickly get up from the lift chair and get to the kitchen. Even if I could get there in time, what I can do from a wheelchair is limited. Also, I couldn't tell her what to do and expect that she could do it. Therefore, I use DoorDash, a food delivery service, or bring home food from restaurants. I also buy Honey Baked Smoked Turkey that will last for several meals. My friend Joel Elmore brings hot roasted chicken from Costco when he goes there. He cuts the breasts off the chicken and slices them up. This and some cranberry sauce can provide two or three meals. Occasionally, I fry hot dogs. I limit this as well because I don't want her to see the stove in use.

She doesn't always remember that I am her husband or that she has children and grandchildren. I use photo albums stored on my computer to show them on the TV screen. Also, I make DVDs and Blu-rays of reunions and vacations that I can show her on the TV. We also have many family pictures around the house. We can pick them up and talk about them.

Since I couldn't drive at that time, I relied on Jodie's friends and Uber to get her to social and religious events. I would watch the progress of Uber until she arrived at her destination. Once a driver decided to drop her off a block away to make it easier for himself. I knew this was a huge problem. Her friend, Colleen Homolka, had moved and Jodie had never been to her new house. I called Colleen, but the call went to voicemail. All cell phones are turned off for these meetings. Then I called Jodie's cell phone, concerned that she frequently doesn't know how to answer it. Luckily, she did this time. I asked her to go to the nearest intersection and tell me the name of the streets. As mentioned earlier, she isn't good at following directions, but I was able to get her close. Fortunately, her friends saw her outside and called to her.

After that, I would only use Uber when she was going to very familiar homes. I also called to her destination, providing the expected arrival time, car description, and driver's name. Still, I would sometimes get calls from the drivers because Jodie would tell them they were not going where they should. Eventually, I had to stop using Uber. That meant that she was dependent on two friends who could sometimes take her. After an incident described later, one of them no longer thought it was safe to drive Jodie. This created a problem for her crucial social life.

The next chapter discusses how I tried to meet Jodie's needs and keep her happy.

28

Potential Solutions

"Too often, we underestimate the power of a touch, a smile, a kind word, a listening ear, an honest compliment, or the smallest act of caring, all of which have the potential to turn a life around."
—Leo Buscaglia, in a 1993 issue of *Reader's Digest*

I knew that Jodie was not at fault for her changed behavior; it was the disease. It was my responsibility to minimize the chances that these situations would occur. It was also vital for me to find ways to make her happy. I needed to find what would change her mood from sadness, anger, depression, disappointment, frustration, or stress to happiness and satisfaction. Listed below are some things that I tried that you might consider as a caregiver. Thoroughly reading the references I have provided, and others, will be beneficial. The National Institute on Aging (NIA)[1] is particularly useful. It has many sources on multiple subjects that will be of interest to you. You won't have to "reinvent the wheel" as I did.

Express Your Love

The most effective and frequent method I use to keep Jodie happy is to tell her how much I love her. This requires no effort from me because I am almost always very happy and just blurt it out many times a day for no particular reason except a desire to say it. Since she feels the same way, she does it too; you would be surprised how often that happens. I also started saying it to help her mood after dementia got more serious, mainly before going out in public.

Music

Music can be a very effective way to help deal with memory issues. My first experience with the power of music was when my sister Ellen Reed had a stroke. When Jodie and I visited her, she couldn't speak a coherent sentence until she was told to sing it. Instantly, she could express herself. I use music with Jodie every day. I can make her happy or change her mood by playing the music she loves. For years, I have known that she loves the McGuire Sisters and other music from the

'50s and '60s. The McGuire Sisters were even mentioned in her description in her high school yearbook. I recorded and kept a PBS TV show that features artists from this timeframe, including the McGuire Sisters. I have also used Pandora and Amazon Echo Dot. However, YouTube videos are the most effective. It is amazing how quickly her mood changes from sadness, depression, or anger to happiness when I play the McGuire Sisters, Andrea Bocelli, André Rieu's concerts, and others. The change is instant and amazing. She gets a broad smile, stands up and starts dancing, singing, or conducting the music. I have found that other music can have a similar effect and change it up for variety. She was an excellent piano player and found a way to deal with stress by playing the piano.

According to an NPR article[2] sent to me by my sister Ellen, studies have shown that music can be used therapeutically with dementia patients to help with cognition, behavior, and mood. The article confirms my observations with Jodie and is a vital strategy I use to help her. The article relates a story about a woman who suffered from dementia and lived in a memory care facility. Her daughter, a former opera singer, found her mother sad and confused. Her mother didn't recognize her and was not communicating. When she started playing the piano and singing, her mother sang with her. Afterward, her mother started joking with her and made a comment that indicated she knew her last name. Jodie hasn't reacted as dramatically as this, but music makes her very happy and is a great mood changer.

For more information on this valuable tool, search articles on Music and Memory.

Optimism and Humor

These traits come naturally to me. Others have told me that I display a positive, optimistic attitude. It has been hard to feel and display these traits in the most difficult times, but I am nearly always happy, optimistic and make Jodie laugh many times each day. One of the themes of this book is that a positive attitude is vital to successfully live with the challenges of progressive disease and other chronic conditions. This is also the case for caregivers. *The Journal of Personality* published an article titled: "The Association Between Actor/Partner Optimism and Cognitive Functioning Among Older Couples."[3] They concluded: "The participant's own optimism and their partner's optimism were both positively associated with cognitive functioning."[4]

Laughter has many benefits for both the caregiver and the patient. Alzheimer's.net has a good article titled "Laughter for Alzheimer's Prevention"[5] that outlines these benefits. They list caregiver benefits as "heart disease prevention, lower stress hormones, ease of anxiety and fear, increase in social interaction, lower blood sugar levels, and strengthened immune system."[6] Patient benefits include "allowing them to redirect negative emotions, easing symptoms of depression, tempering signs of aggression, reducing stress, and improving social interaction."[7]

Exercise

For many years my wife and I took long walks. These were relaxing, fun times when we would talk about upcoming events and memories from the past. Even after I was using a motorized scooter or wheelchair, we would take "walks." This was healthy for Jodie because she got good exercise as well as a stress reliever. It was time for us to be together and enjoy each other's company. We were very happy and always expressed our love for each other. The California weather made it possible to do this all year.

This is what HelpGuide has to say about exercise: "Exercise is one of the best stress-relievers for both the Alzheimer's patient and you, the caregiver.... [It] ... can have a positive effect on many problem behaviors, such as aggression, wandering, and difficulty sleeping."[8]

Animals

Lisa Reed, my daughter-in-law, read that animals can be beneficial to people with dementia because they want to take care of something. This is certainly true with my wife, Jodie, who even tries to give away her food to other people at our table at restaurants. She's always trying to take care of other people. But we are not in a position to take care of a pet. Knowing this, Lisa found a Hasbro companion dog that is battery-operated. It can move its head, wag its tail, blink its eyes and make barking sounds. You can turn it on for both sound and movement, movement only, or no action. At first, Jodie was fascinated but then wanted to give it food and drink. She worried about it urinating on the rug and insisted that it was a real animal. At times, she even thought it was a real person, one who was so young we couldn't go for a walk and leave it alone. She sometimes spent so much time taking care of it that it seemed a burden to her and wanted me to take it. After a while, I turned off sound and movement. That worked better.

My sister Ellen bought Jodie a stuffed dog that is smaller and doesn't weigh as much as it has no electronics inside. Jodie's favorite varies from time to time between the Hasbro dog or the stuffed dog. I had some concerns about how much time she devoted to them. She was no longer watching the news or interacting with me as frequently. I started making the dogs disappear for a time each day and reappear when it seemed appropriate. This procedure worked pretty well.

While there were some unexpected results, the overall impact of these companion dogs has been great. Both have had a very positive effect on my wife. She spends a lot of time petting and talking with each one. Jodie generally became much happier, and the stress in the house is dramatically reduced now that we have the dogs. There is some confusion in her mind about whether the dogs are real or not. As I have never been willing to lie to her, I explain that they are companion dogs that do certain things, but they are not alive, so they can't eat, drink or go to the bathroom. While she hears this, she still believes they are real, and I don't press the point.

Fred Hellrich, a fraternity brother, related a story to me about the positive reaction patients have to dogs. While his wife, Mary Hellrich, was temporarily in a nursing home recovering from the after-effects of surgery, Fred took their dog on his daily visits. Here are his comments: "The facility allowed (even encouraged) it, and had many visitors that would bring their therapy dogs to visit the residents. For me, I had to stop and spend a few minutes with any of the residents that happened to be in the hallways on my way in. It could take me 15 minutes to get to Mary's room. But the residents really did appreciate it. It was wonderful to see how they just lit up when I came in. It didn't take long for all of them to know 'Sandy's' name. Sandy is a rescue dog that we had DNA tested to determine her breed. Her primary breeds are Golden Retriever, Labrador Retriever and Border Collie. She would be a perfect therapy dog. In fact, her trainer suggested that we get her certified for it."

If you can care for a dog, there are service dogs that can perform numerous helpful tasks. I recommend an article from Alzheimer's Universe titled "Can Specially Trained Dogs Help People with Alzheimer's Dementia?"[9] Below are some brief excerpts from this article:

> Only a few breeds qualify to be trained as dementia service dogs including, Labrador and Golden Retrievers, German Shepherds and Border Collies.... Dementia service dogs respond to sound triggers in the home. For example, an electronic timer triggers a sound that can alert the dog to bring a bag of medicine to the owner.... The service dog is also trained to respond to special instructions, such as the "home" command.... Service dogs can ... trigger an alarm for emergency situations.[10]

My research indicates that pets can reduce stress, anxiety, and depression. Pets show unconditional love and bring joy to their owner. As they need to walk, patients can get the exercise that they might not otherwise have gotten.

Because we couldn't own a dog, I looked into organizations that offer pet visits for people in our situation where an animal would be helpful part-time. Other more serious difficulties arose about that time, so we didn't take advantage of that option, but you might want to consider it.

Pictures and Videos

As mentioned earlier, there were a few methods I used to remind Jodie of important people and events and to keep her happy. I took a lot of pictures and videos of family reunions and vacations from which I made DVDs and Blu-rays. When she forgot she had kids or grandkids, I would show her pictures or play a video. We also have framed pictures around the house as well as photo albums that she can peruse. The NIA recommends: "Keep well-loved objects and photographs around the house to help the person feel more secure."[11]

Other Suggestions

The references I have provided offer other suggestions and caregiving tips that I have not used. I might have to use them later, and they might be useful to you. An example relates to napping. Mayo Clinic recommends that you limit napping so that your patient doesn't confuse day and night. This recommendation is entirely logical, and you should follow it if you can. However, as I mentioned earlier, there are things the experts recommend that just aren't possible in my situation. You will probably find the same. Even before Jodie had memory loss, she always napped by falling asleep while watching television during the day, early evening, and late at night. However, she was still able to get a full night's sleep. If I were to try to stop her from napping, it would cause stress and conflict. Occasionally she does so much napping that she is up early in the morning. Fortunately, when I tell her I need more sleep, she usually goes back to bed. Based on a lot of experience caring for her, I judge that it is much better to let her nap and avoid the conflict that would result from trying to stop her. Your situation could be very different.

Notwithstanding my comment that some recommendations found in the references might not work for you, I repeat my suggestion that you thoroughly review the resources I have provided. For example, in the NIH National Institute on Aging, you will find links on a page and, after selecting one, will find that it has links to still more pages. The result is a great number of useful resources.

A sampling of topics, some of which I have not covered in detail, follows:

Coping with Agitation and Aggression in Alzheimer's Disease
When a Person with Alzheimer's Rummages and Hides Things[*]
Wandering and Alzheimer's Disease[†]
Alzheimer's and Hallucinations, Delusions, and Paranoia
Tips for Coping with Sundowning[‡]
Managing Personality and Behavior Changes in Alzheimer's
Prepare for the road ahead: Who will make healthcare and/or financial
    decisions? Where will your loved one live?[§]

Accelerated Decline

The solutions I used worked well for years. However, in July 2019, the situation changed. Jodie rapidly declined, which led to a real crisis that would greatly affect our lives. This is the subject of the next chapter.

---

   [*] I never found a fully satisfactory solution but did have some hiding places that helped.
   [†] I will address this in Chapter 32: Initial Accommodations, Serious Threats.
   [‡] Sundowner's syndrome or sundowning occurs in dementia patients around twilight. It can involve confusion, agitation, and sadness. Some patients even experience delusions or hallucinations. It is distressing for patients and challenging for caregivers. Jodie has a mild form of Sundowner's some evenings. I make sure she is happy at that time of the day to minimize or avoid Sundowner's.
   [§] I address aspects of this throughout this section.

29

The Crisis

Big Problems, Out of Answers

"The caregiver's journey ... does not proceed from stage to stage in a neat fashion.
It is definitely not linear. It feels like we are going around in circles thinking we have resolved a crisis only to have it return or be superseded by a different, unexpected crisis."
—Gail Sheehy, in *Passages in Caregiving: Turning Chaos into Confidence* (2011)

In July 2019, it became clear that Jodie's rapid decline was going to change our lives. We attended an annual Reed reunion, and her behavior was very negative at times, mainly when there was a large group. We were able to manage it somewhat by playing music by the McGuire Sisters.

I had read that being among large groups of strangers can increase stress for Alzheimer's patients, whereas interactions with smaller groups have the opposite impact.* We weren't among strangers, but due to Jodie's memory loss, they seemed to be strangers to her.

After the reunion, other symptoms, like non-compliance and incontinence, got worse. But my inability to join my friends for lunch or ever leave her alone pushed me over the edge into crisis mode. I was overwhelmed and seemed to have no answers regarding how to help her. I knew that being her caregiver now had to be a full-time job and that I could not do this alone.

For a person who always felt like he was in control of his life, finding that you're not in control is very disconcerting. I laid awake at night trying to see a way to deal with the situation. Seeing none, at times, I broke down and started crying in bed. At lunch with my friends, I broke down as well. On some phone calls, I choked up. I made sure this never happened in front of Jodie.

I had to renew my efforts to get Jodie some medication despite her reluctance even to take vitamins. Also, I had to find caregivers to give me some relief. This would also be challenging due to her aversion to having people in the house. I believed that if I could accomplish these things, the situation

---

* As I will explain in Chapter 30, the senior living facility is more conducive to one-on-one social interactions.

would be manageable again. If I couldn't, our ability to live in our home and my ability to care for Jodie without having a nervous breakdown myself would be impossible. I pursued both objectives simultaneously but will discuss them separately.

Caregivers

Our medical conditions and the fact that neither of us could drive significantly affected my social life. It devolved to lunch once a week with my golf friends when my friend John Wyatt could drive me. Beyond that, my only social life was an occasional lunch with my neighbor, Steve Steen. These times were critical to my well-being. They were the only times I could be away from caregiving responsibilities. It doesn't matter how much you love someone and enjoy being with them; you need to have some time to yourself and time to enjoy the company of others. The only time I could be by myself was when Jodie went to Renew. Even then, some of those occasions had to be spent with my handyman. As stated before, Jodie hates having people in the house who are not friends or relatives. Even that can be a problem if they stay overnight. She reacts negatively if they go into her room. However, it is her room that is often a gigantic mess that needs to be cleaned.

All manner of things can be under the bed, on top of the bed, and between the sheets and blankets. Often this includes essential items of mine that are missing. Sometimes clutter on her bed is a couple of feet high. The nightstand, desk, and dresser are also cluttered. Drawers are stuffed with paper and miscellaneous things. The floor is littered with shoes. Also, she hides things under the bed that I need to find but can't myself. I have to take advantage of the opportunity to clean up her room when I can. Because of Jodie's reaction to Tom Busta, our handyman, he likes to come when she is at Renew and finish before she returns.

I don't have to worry about her when she is with friends but do when I am with mine. The approach I used was to make her happy by playing music well before I left to ensure she was in a good mood. I posted lists of all the people she might want to call in plain sight in several places. I taped down index cards with my cell number and 911 on the end table by the phone. As I left, I set it up so she would have her favorite music playing while I was gone. I called her when I got to the restaurant, during lunch, and when I left for home.

This process eventually started to fail. Once, when I called during lunch, she was in a near panic because she couldn't find me. She didn't remember that I went to lunch and didn't think to call me. On another occasion, I got a call from Heather Elmore, one of her friends, who told me that Jodie had called her and was very scared. A man came to the house and tried to get in. Heather tried to calm her by telling her it was probably Tim Heck, our contractor, who was working in the house. I called and calmed her down but needed to leave the restaurant earlier than planned.

I knew then that my options were to hire some caregivers or have no social life. No social life would have been very unhealthy for me. That, in turn, would not be good for Jodie. Luckily, Terry Totten, one of my wife's friends, knew two people who could be part-time caregivers. One was a friend of hers who lives a short walk from us, and the other was a cousin. Both had been associated with professional caregiving organizations, one owned her own caregiving company. They were both willing to come as needed, if they were available, and did not require a minimum number of days or hours per week. I couldn't believe my luck. They seemed ideal, particularly Terry's friend who could walk to our house and had good availability.

I was concerned about how well this would work because Jodie is miserable and anxious anytime people are in our home. I decided to utilize both of the caregivers. Jodie was not very receptive to either of them, but I knew that I could not handle the situation without their help. I just made it clear to her that they were going to be there regularly. She was not happy with that but accepted it for a while. The two caregivers referred to us should have been less of a problem in this regard because of their relationship with Terry. Not being here regularly would also help.

Unfortunately, my optimism was not well-founded. From the outset, Jodie did not "like" them. It was only a few weeks before one of them resigned. She had good reasons. In one case, I had her take Jodie to lunch with the Renew group which follows the Renew meeting. But this time, only one other girl was going to lunch, and the caregiver was driving both of them. None of Jodie's closest friends went to lunch that day. Jodie demanded to go home, but the caregiver knew I had the handyman at home and wanted Jodie out of the house, so she tried to talk Jodie out of it.

As I understand it, Jodie jumped out of the car when they stopped and started through a parking lot. The caregiver thought this was dangerous and called to tell me she felt she had to bring Jodie home. I talked to Jodie briefly and agreed. In another incident, Jodie told the caregiver to get out of the house. When she didn't, Jodie got up in her face and said: "Why are you still here? I told you to get out!" Then she started throwing things … a typical reaction when she is mad. She didn't throw anything at the caregiver but it was very disturbing to her.

The caregiver knew how badly I needed her and wanted to help. Nevertheless, it was untenable for her, and she wasn't helping Jodie. She had to quit. The other caregiver was less available and undoubtedly heard these stories because the caregivers knew each other. These stories caused one of Jodie's friends to tell me that she could no longer drive Jodie to Renew. She has a medical condition and it would be dangerous if Jodie was upset and bumped her. She loves Jodie and was crying when she told me.

I considered using professional caregivers like Visiting Angels but, from prior research and interviews with them, knew that they would require a minimum number of days a week and a minimum number of hours per visit. Given Jodie's aversion to having strangers in the house, this would never work. It would entail much more intrusion than the two caregivers and Jodie had rejected them adamantly.

Good caregivers were one of the two solutions I hoped would allow us to stay in our home. It failed with ominous implications.

Medication

Now my only hope was medication. What a long shot! Getting Jodie to go to a doctor was a challenge. Having the right medication prescribed would not be easy either. Then, how was I going to get her to take medicine? Even if successful on those counts, would medication return her behavior close to the unusually fantastic person that she was? This disease changes personality; medication was unlikely to undo much about that. I am resourceful, pride myself on being an optimist with a positive attitude, and am a problem solver. I am also a pragmatist, so I knew that finding a satisfactory solution to this set of challenges was really going to test me. I intended to push hard, doing whatever could be done to get the right medication prescribed and taken. However, even if successful, more radical decisions would probably have to be made without caregivers' help.

I decided to work on both issues in parallel. I would try to get a near-term appointment with a neurologist and also find a way to deliver the medication. Many of our friends have had to care for parents or friends who had dementia or Alzheimer's disease. I learned from them that the antipsychotic drugs were not helpful in their cases, but anti-anxiety drugs were. They told me that their observations of Jodie indicated to them that she needed anti-anxiety drugs. I felt the same way for a long time because I could see how anxious she got about the gardeners outside, the trash collectors, and people that came into the house, e.g., contractors, handyman and cleaning personnel. Getting anti-anxiety medication was my goal.

The neurologist that I used to get Medicare approval for my wheelchair had left the practice after a brief period. Once again, we had to get a new neurologist. I thought the fastest way to do this was to get one from the same practice. A helpful neurologist responded to a plea I made via their message system. After listening to my explanation of the situation, he decided to give us a near-term appointment with the first available neurologist. That turned out to be a lady who would retire at the end of the year. I was disappointed that we couldn't have him, but we needed help immediately. I knew Jodie wouldn't go to the doctor if she understood it was for her, so I told her that it was an appointment for us. That was true. I needed to help her but also to have the ability to care for her and have a happy life myself.

While I was waiting for the neurologist appointment and a prescription, I explored methods of delivering the drugs. Through Internet research, I found that even a severe psychiatric patient that is a danger to themselves and others can, with a court order, be held in a hospital. Still, they cannot be given medicine without their consent.

Like every other challenge that I have run into with my situation, I sought an answer. I contacted my attorney and explained the situation to him. He told me that there was a way to deal with this, which is called a conservatorship. This represents an approach to deal with one of the topics covered in the National Institute on Aging that I referenced earlier, namely, "Who will make healthcare and/ or financial decisions?"[1] It needed to be me in the near-term, but a successor or successors also needed to be established. The other solution, Medical Power of Attorney, is discussed in detail later in this section.

Generally, conservatorships are granted for people who have advanced Alzheimer's disease or other serious illnesses or injuries. Conservators are appointed by a judge and have the authority to manage the affairs of those no longer capable of making rational decisions about finances or health care. A Conservator of the Estate takes care of financial matters only. A Conservator of the Person takes care of both medical and personal decisions. There are significant drawbacks to conservatorships. They usually require court hearings and the ongoing assistance of a lawyer. They are time-consuming and expensive. The conservator must keep detailed records and file court papers regularly. The court proceedings and documents are in the public record and represent an intrusion into one's independence and privacy. I didn't have the time or desire to pursue this as a solution.

I had already addressed the financial decision situation months earlier. I told my estate attorney that my wife was no longer able to function as a trustee of our living trust. However, I feared that she would not be willing to sign the paperwork due to her aversion to signing anything. A good example is that I needed her to sign a legal document that would grant us a large sum of money. It took a lot of time and persuasion to accomplish this. The estate attorney advised me to get a letter from my GP who knew her medical situation stating that she was not capable of making financial decisions.

My GP wrote the following letter that enabled me to change the trustee from my wife to my son.

> I am the primary care physician for Joan Reed. She has been my patient for 7 years. In my medical opinion, Mrs. Reed suffers from dementia, which has progressed to a point where she no longer has the capacity to handle her finances. Likewise, I believe she is unable to administer a trust or fulfill similar responsibilities. I do not expect her condition to improve.

However, this didn't cover medical decisions. I needed a Conservator of Person. To get a conservatorship decision, you have to go to court. Also, you need a qualified doctor to certify the condition of the patient. This was the second reason for getting an appointment with the neurologist.

There was another solution. If I could get signed durable powers of attorney for finances and health care designating me, my son or daughter to make such decisions, we wouldn't need a conservator. We could take charge. There was one more step. A doctor had to certify that Jodie was not capable of making these decisions. We hoped to get this from the neurologist. Unfortunately, as previously mentioned, getting Jodie to sign documents of any kind, even those involving significant financial benefit, is nearly impossible. I did not believe I would have any chance of getting her to sign a power of attorney.

If you haven't already done so, I strongly recommend that you execute durable powers of attorney for health care, powers of attorney for financial matters, a living trust with successor trustees, advance health care directives, authorizations to release health information protected by the Health Insurance Portability & Accountability Act (HIPAA), and conventional wills while both parties are mentally competent. Hire an estate attorney who knows the laws in your state.

Given the immediate need for medication, my conclusion was that if I couldn't convince her to take it, I would have to find a way to give it to her. I had not gone through the process of becoming a conservator, nor was it clear whether that would allow me to give her medication without her consent. So a consequential decision had to be made.

I decided to do what some friends had advised me to do long ago, crush the medicine and put it in food or drink. My answer had always been that there were legal implications, but I was more concerned about losing her trust. I don't lie to anybody, certainly not Jodie. If she realized I did that, I could lose her trust, which could change our relationship. With her condition, lying to her would often make her feel better, but I don't do it. I find ways to avoid it, like changing the subject. I felt that giving her medicine was akin to lying.

Nevertheless, I decided that getting her medication was so essential and immediate that I would have to do it. I would continue to seek a legal solution that granted me the authority to give her medicine and make medical decisions in the future. Our children strongly supported this decision. Once again, I was warned that some people might decide to make trouble for me about this. My opinion, and my son's, was similar to the reaction we had concerning my method of stopping Jodie's violence. I had to do what was best for Jodie and be candid with my readers, regardless of the potential consequences for me.

Before we met the neurologist, I sent a long message to her describing the situation and asked whether we could have a brief one-on-one before she saw Jodie. Things went south right away! The neurologist did briefly meet with me but her attitude was very negative. I got the distinct impression that she viewed me as an overly controlling husband. At the outset, she said: "I can't treat her if she won't take medicine." I told her that I was working with an attorney on a conservatorship. Her response was "That won't help. You still can't give her medicine without her consent." I told her that recently she had taken medicine from me. That was true. It was also true that this was rare and was Tylenol for headaches.

She provided a diagnosis of "severe dementia and I suspect she has Alzheimer's disease." She wanted blood and other tests to confirm Alzheimer's, but I knew getting those tests would be impossible. Unfortunately, the neurologist did not prescribe an anti-anxiety drug. She prescribed an antipsychotic medicine, Quetiapine.

I had previously decided to crush the medication and put it in her morning orange juice. While not explicitly explaining what I was doing, I would do everything in front of Jodie. Splitting the medicine or crushing would be done in front of her. So would putting the pill fragments in the glass. I openly discussed the name of her medication, medication type and dosage to people in person and on phone calls with her near me. She has heard me talk to the pharmacy while giving her name, birth date, and medication name multiple times. What does she know and understand about this? I don't know and don't ask. As one of my friends said to me: "Who is going to complain?" My main concern was the possibility that giving her medication could seriously harm her. I don't think I could handle that or ever get over it even though I would be following the doctor's instructions.

The medication seemed to have a very negative effect almost immediately. Jodie started talking gibberish about 30 minutes after she took it. She had a severe headache and said she felt sick. This is what I feared! I laid awake worrying that, by giving her the medication, I had harmed her. I was hoping that the effects would not be permanent because I had read that some could be. I stopped the medication after two alarming days. I then found this on Drugs.com[2]: "There is a higher chance of death in older adults who take this medicine (quetiapine tablets) for mental problems caused by dementia…. This medicine is not approved to treat mental problems caused by dementia."

I tried to get the neurologist to prescribe an anti-anxiety medication instead of another antipsychotic or, if necessary, in addition to an antipsychotic. Instead, she prescribed another antipsychotic. I kept increasing the dose as prescribed but could see no positive effect. It appeared at times that it had a negative impact. The neurologist had no interest in my observations and just said: "It's not the medication; it's the disease." Then I asked to meet with the neurologist that we would use after her retirement for a second opinion. She absolutely refused to allow this. From prior discussions with him, before she was assigned to us, I was confident that he would prescribe anti-anxiety medication.

It is very important to find doctors that you have confidence in, and who will listen to and respond to your concerns. We didn't have that. I didn't tell the neurologist that she was fired, but I was done with her. I discontinued that medicine by removing it slowly, decreasing the dosage over time until Jodie was completely off it.

I was stymied. I didn't trust the neurologist. She was not willing to listen to my concerns, would not prescribe anti-anxiety drugs, and would not let me talk to the doctor who would become the permanent neurologist until he took over. At this point, I had failed to achieve both of my objectives. I had no caregivers and no effective medication. Once again, I was overwhelmed and without answers.

I very reluctantly concluded that we could no longer live in our home under present conditions, and I couldn't change them. The next chapter describes the options considered and the decisions made.

30

Senior Living Decision Rationale

"Not all storms come to disrupt your life, some come to clear your path."

—Anonymous

The Decision Process

Even before the events of July 2019 that pushed me into crisis mode, I had realized that our living conditions would eventually have to change. I thought the time would come when Jodie would need to be placed into a memory care facility but had assumed that would be in the distant future. At that time, there had seemed to be several options. Jodie's rapid decline eliminated most of them. I still want to share my decision process with you in case your situation is different. Here are three of the scenarios I considered, the steps taken to implement them, and why each proved unsuitable for us.

Scenario 1

When it became necessary to put Jodie into memory care, I would find a facility near our home in California. Then I could take her to the facility each night, bring her home in the morning, and spend the day with her. That way, she could get the care she needed, be able to enjoy our home, and still see her friends. I would have some relief from constant caregiving and could spend some time with my friends without worrying about her.

I visited two places in Danville, California, and had brochures for other nearby facilities. This was an attractive concept in many respects but soon was not a viable option. To ensure that Jodie would have family close by if I were to die first, my long-range plan was to relocate to Phoenix, Arizona, where our son's family lives. At the rate Jodie's mental condition was declining, that long-range plan needed to be implemented in the near-term.

I had to eliminate this option. If your circumstances are different and you already live near your family, you might consider a plan similar to this.

Scenario 2

We could buy a second home in Phoenix. That would be consistent with our long-range plan. We would live in Arizona part-time. We would stay there for a few weeks at a time to start a longer-term transition to Arizona. That way we could maintain the social interactions that my wife and I had with our friends in California, which were very important to us. I didn't want those relationships to atrophy by long absences. Besides, we were both delighted with our house, grounds, and location. I believed that a dramatic change from that situation would not be good for either of us. It was not likely that we would make many new friends in a new location at our age and condition.

In July, the revelation I had about the care required for Jodie proved that I couldn't get the support I needed in California. It wasn't rational to think that we could continue to live in our home in California, even part of the year. We needed to implement the long-range plan of moving to Arizona as soon as possible ... much sooner than I had hoped. Our permanent home would have to be in Arizona.

This concept of owning a second home could be ideal for those with the financial means, who have no restrictions regarding travel, and are not dealing with progressive disease. Unfortunately, this is not the case for us. Traveling is problematic, and we both have progressive diseases.

Scenario 3

Another option considered was buying a house in Arizona and live there full-time. We would not sell our California house for two reasons. The house is a valuable asset; selling it would incur significant taxation. Capital gains tax could be avoided or minimized by having the house pass to the estate. If I were the one left behind, I would have the opportunity to live again in our California home.

The goal was to find a home close to our son's home and was on a golf course to have great views and attractive landscaping. Our son's home is on a golf course, so if we found a house on the same course, it would be possible to be close to his house and have such views. Finding a place meeting those objectives would allow us to get help from the family. We would be able to enjoy being with family during holidays as well as birthdays. This only happened once or twice a year while we lived in California.

We engaged a real estate agent in early August 2019 to find a home that would meet our objectives and accommodate my physical limitations. We looked at several homes suggested to us by our agent and found a beautiful home on a golf course with great views. A great advantage was that it would be an easy walk to our son's house. It also seemed to be under the market price. It seemed ideal. However, it was clear that we would have to make major modifications to the home. All the doors would have to be widened, and one room had a step-down floor that would have to be elevated.

The biggest problem was the bathroom layout. It would be impossible for me to shower without substantial modifications, which would include, among other things, moving the wall between the master bedroom and the bathroom at significant expense. Having looked at many other homes, it was evident that all the homes available would require major, expensive modifications. Such expenditure was unjustified for what could be a short-term solution.

The strong desire to retain our independence and live in a home that met all our goals clouded rational thinking and prevented me from seeing the obvious. Considering our progressively debilitating conditions, it was unclear how long this or any other house would work for us. Even if we found the perfect home that didn't require expensive modifications, at best, it would be only a temporary solution. Most likely, a home of our own would not be adequate. We needed more care than we would be able to get, even with our family's help.

I realized that if Jodie passed before me, I would not return to California. Living in that big house alone would bring back too many memories. As my diseases progressed, I would need family and other support as well.

If you are not dealing with progressive diseases, moving near your family and modifying a home to meet your needs could be a rational decision; it wasn't for us.

None of the above options were suitable for our situation. We needed to move into a senior living facility that offered independent living, assisted living, and memory care to avoid moving again and get the help we needed.

Choosing a Care Facility

I was no longer capable of managing everything on my own. Moving into a care facility would make our life simpler. Relative to the size of our home in California, we would be living in a small apartment. Caring for a much smaller apartment would be considerably easier than caring for our four-bedroom house. Once a week, housekeeping would clean the unit, including making the beds and changing the sheets. Most of our meals would be prepared by the dining room in the facility or restaurants nearby. Not making meals would mean much less food shopping and dishwashing. We would have a closer family life and more physical support from our family than we could get in California.

Through the efforts of our son, Mike, and daughter-in-law, Lisa, we found a senior care facility called LivGenerations Ahwatukee. It was about eight miles from their home and had independent living, assisted living and memory care. The facility was only three years old and resembled a resort. The best apartment in the facility was available. It looked over a courtyard and was on the first floor. We would have to decide quickly because the apartment was very desirable, and others were interested.

I had to resolve two major challenges. First, I had to satisfy myself that the apartment would work for us, considering my disabilities. Second, I had to get effective medication to deal with Jodie's anxieties before we moved, something I had failed to accomplish earlier. If we found that LivGenerations would work for us, we would want to reserve the apartment quickly before it was no longer available. That would leave only four or five weeks before we moved to Arizona. Preparing for the move, the two-day trip to Arizona, moving into a temporary apartment while we waited for the moving van, transferring to the permanent apartment, and adjusting to living in a senior care facility would be very stressful for Jodie. I needed to get anti-anxiety medication for her as soon as possible. As it takes a while before medication builds up in the system, we needed medication before the move for it to be effective. Without proper medication, the process of moving would be a disaster.

Deciding Whether LivGenerations Would Work

I had to make sure that the apartment would accommodate my wheelchair, commode, and shower chair. I needed to be able to transfer to the commode. I also needed to be able to transfer to the shower chair and be able to maneuver the shower chair into the shower.

In my home, the shower chair functioned as both the commode and the shower chair. However, it was clear from the apartment's layout that I would need a separate, fixed-position commode due to space restrictions in the master bath. Fortunately, the travel commode I owned would serve that purpose. Two significant issues remained to be solved. What furniture and equipment would fit in the apartment without restricting wheelchair maneuvering? Would it be possible to shower with my specialized equipment in the relatively small master bathroom?

Fortunately, Fred Hellrich, one of my fraternity brothers, told me about the National Association of Senior and Specialty Move Managers, an organization that helps seniors relocate. He provided a link* to the organization, which allowed me to find two move manager companies near me, one of which was in my town.

The all-encompassing contract that both firms offered was not acceptable because I knew I would have a certain amount of help from my handyman, friends, neighbors, and family. I wasn't sure what I would need from the move manager other than a layout of the apartment with furnishings. I negotiated a contract with Cassy Eriksson, the move manager in my town, wherein I initially authorized the apartment layout. Any additional scope would have to be approved in writing.

She modified her contract and decided that she would use the modified contract for all future clients. She turned out to be spectacularly helpful. I added to the scope as time went on. For example, we left a day before the moving van came. I had no concerns about having Cassy manage the movers in my absence.

LivGenerations provided basic dimensions. Our son and daughter-in-law augmented the basic information with more details. Cassy measured all the items I wanted to take and created several layouts that allowed me to decide what I could and couldn't take. These layouts eliminated some items I wanted but

---

* https://www.nasmm.org/find/index.cfm.

ensured that I could maneuver everywhere I needed to go. The best design was found through an iterative process that included suggestions from our son, Mike, and me. It was a reasonable result considering the limitations of a smaller facility.

However, it wasn't clear that I could shower, considering that I use a wheelchair and need to transfer to the shower chair. Then I have to be able to get the shower chair into the shower. To find out, the move manager made cutouts to scale of the shower chair and the wheelchair. That allowed us to move them around to try various options. We found one that appeared to work if LivGenerations would remove a shower bench. The solution's uncertainty was a little disconcerting, but based on the issues we found when house hunting, this was the best situation I was likely to find. Even if our plan didn't work, I had always found solutions for problems that came up in the past, so showering was not a deal-breaker. We signed a contract to move into the apartment of our choice in LivGenerations.

Medication

I talked to our niece, Julie Bowman, a nurse practitioner, to get some guidance on how to provide the medication that Jodie needed. She said that behavioral health medication with dementia patients over 65 involves trial and error, so you need a provider who is willing to listen to feedback. She suggested that I find a psychiatrist specializing in senior behavioral health because they tend to be more empathetic than neurologists. She thought anti-anxiety medication would be helpful and mentioned that Lexapro and Celexa could help with anxiety. Her direct experience was some years ago, but patients with dementia and aggressive behaviors often had Ativan ordered on an as-needed basis. Because of the side effects, it is usually not a scheduled medication. She thought it could be used if Jodie's behaviors were so severe that I was concerned for her safety or when she needed medical treatment.

I got a referral from our GP to a psychiatrist. Fortunately, we got an early appointment. He prescribed Celexa, an anti-anxiety medication. Years earlier, the neurologist we had most trusted suggested Celexa for Jodie, but Jodie wasn't willing to take it. Celexa was also the medication my friends recommended and one our niece suggested.

We got the prescription about two weeks before the move and started the lower dose her doctor recommended immediately. Before the move, I increased the dosage to a higher level as directed by the doctor. The effect was immediate and noticed by everyone. Her friends noticed that Jodie was much better. Our family was amazed at the improvement. As a result, the move went far better than expected. It helped immensely that our daughter, Kris, made the trip from California to Arizona with us and stayed a while.

The following chapter describes the challenges we faced to implement the move to LivGenerations and how they were overcome.

31

The Challenges of Moving to Senior Living

"Alone, we can do so little; together we can do so much."
—Helen Keller

Preparing for the Move

I can't adequately explain the extreme challenge I faced to move us from a large four-bedroom home into a much smaller two-bedroom apartment in a time frame of four or five weeks. It would be challenging for anyone. But the difficulty of accomplishing it with my handicaps, the time caregiving consumes, plus the fact that Jodie couldn't help and would likely complicate matters made it look like an impossible challenge. But many factors combined to make it possible.

Over 53 years of marriage, we had accumulated too many things. When people move, they have an excellent opportunity to get rid of things they don't need. We lived in our California home for 34 years so we hadn't done that for a long time. With only two people living in a four-bedroom house, it was too easy to keep things. There was an enormous quantity of items that we couldn't take to Arizona. Since we weren't going to sell the house, much of it could be behind. My family encouraged me to do just that because of the enormity of the task and my physical limitations.

Two considerations caused me to ignore that good advice. By now, I knew I would never come back and didn't want my family to have to deal with the task of disposing of things when they sold the house. (You will see the same philosophy in Appendices III and IV regarding end-of-life planning.) Also, I thought it would complicate matters with the movers if there were so many things that were not going mixed in with so many that were. A good example is my walk-in bedroom closet. The floor was covered with all manner of things as were the shelves. Both sides and the end were packed with clothing.

I wanted, and achieved, a closet with nothing on the floor or the shelves. Everything hanging in the closet was going to Arizona. Deciding what to take was time-consuming and depressing. A great majority had to be eliminated. Many favorite shirts and several that had never been worn were discarded. This was true for all items in the house, e.g., clothing, electronics, books, dishes, pans, silverware, pictures, tools, chairs, and many other things. I made all the decisions but got some help from my sister, Ellen, and my daughter, Kris, on Jodie's clothing. I needed an enormous amount of help to execute these decisions and got it as explained below. To reduce Jodie's stress, my friend, George, bought and built wardrobes and put them in the garage. We surreptitiously put the clothing we were taking for her to Arizona in them. Otherwise, she would have gotten upset and returned the clothing she liked to her room.

The volume of things that left the house was massive. I was delighted that other people would benefit from our discards. I gave our cleaning lady and her helper the first choice of charity items. They were thrilled to get them. She was emotional about our leaving and hugged me. My helpers also got some valuable items as well. The rest went to charity.

One suggestion for my readers. Don't wait until you are moving to discard items. If you decide to move, it will make your move much more manageable. If your heirs have to sell your home or clean out your apartment, they will be pleased that you did so.

Aside from the decision-making, my primary contribution was to create an extensive color-coded spreadsheet listing everything in our house that we might want in the apartment. It was a comprehensive spreadsheet that included the following:

1. The item
2. The location where it would go in the apartment
3. Moving van transportation items
4. Personal vehicle transportation items
5. Items to be purchased in Arizona
6. The dimensions of the item
7. Comments about the item
8. Location of the item in California
9. Box number of packed items
10. Contents of that box

The rows listed the items, e.g., juice glasses. The comments column might say how many and which ones. Items in each room were listed in a separate block of rows. The rows were color-coded to indicate those going, those going if they fit in the apartment, those that would be nice to have but were a lower priority, those packed to go, and those not going. As we learned more about the apartment, the color-coding changed. I know this is a lot of detail, but I include it because it might help if you have to make a similar quick move.

In Chapter 5: Build Your Essential Help Network, I discussed the need for a support network that included family, friends, neighbors, a contractor, a handyman, a gardener, and a house-cleaner. When I wrote that chapter, I meant that this support was needed to help you with daily living. I had no idea how critical it would be to execute a major move in a limited time frame.

Once I knew who was willing to help and when they were available, I created an action plan for the individuals who provided help, which I updated daily. My helpers were:

1. Tim Heck, my contractor, who found time in his busy schedule to lower the threshold and widen the door from the kitchen to the garage. I had to go to and from the garage many times a day while preparing for the move. To do that safely, I needed those changes done quickly.

2. Tom Busta, my handyman, who cleared his schedule to make himself as available as possible. I have used him for many years. He is extremely efficient, came when I needed him, and worked long hours. When he was my only helper, he would bring things to me, get my decision and dispose of the items. Using the same example of the closet, he would take an item out of the closet. I would decide to trash it, recycle it, give it to charity or send it to Arizona. He had boxes or laundry baskets for each category and would toss them in the appropriate container. When they were full, he would take them to the garage or driveway for disposition. Tom took away trash, recycle items, and charity items in his vehicle. He also made trips to dispose of hazardous waste.

3. George Homolka, a friend, who is very organized. All I needed to do was tell him that day's objective. He just went off and accomplished the task. He would only interact with me when he needed a decision. Even then, he would accumulate his questions to minimize my time because I was supervising multiple people simultaneously. He often suggested ways to organize things, e.g., locating specific garage areas for various categories of items. I can't tell you how many days he came over and worked for four or five hours. When I learned that the movers would not remove the TV from the wall mount, he and my neighbor Steve removed both the TV and the wall mounting hardware. George removed the stereo equipment from the entertainment center and the computer and accessories from my office desk. He carried away trash, recycle items, and charity items and disposed of them for me. George bought and constructed boxes, including wardrobes.

4. Ellen, my sister, who flew out from Pennsylvania to help for one week. She did a fantastic amount of work, primarily in the kitchen and living room. She pushed me to jettison things, which I needed to do.

5. Steve Steen, a neighbor, who came many days for hours. He was even more extreme than Ellen in terms of strongly encouraging me to toss things.

6. Sara and Mark Ericson, our other neighbors who loaded their cars and their pickup several times to remove a tremendous amount of trash, recyclables, and charity items without being asked. They found a place that would accept anything. That company would sell what they could and send the rest to Bangladesh or somewhere. I was unaware of this company. It was a good choice near the end of the move. Sara and Mark

made at least two trips there. The volume of things they took away was pretty amazing.

7. Kris, our daughter, who came one week early and helped on weekends and evenings. She worked in a remote office that week near our home. One of her many jobs was to pack for Jodie.

8. Mike, our son, who spent the final weekend completing many last-minute tasks.

9. Lisa, our daughter-in-law, who drove over an hour to take my van back to Mobility Works so the instructor's brake could be removed.

10. My golf group who came over several times to bring lunch and offer advice.

The description above about the amazing amount of help that we got doesn't do it justice. Our Senior Move Manager, Cassy, and others who observed it said that it was an incredible thing to watch. We could not have done it without that level of help. I know our helpers realized that and applied the amount of time and effort that they knew was necessary. I can't thank them enough!

Some of Jodie's friends came to say goodbye and to give Jodie a picture of the Renew group. The strength of the relationships we developed with neighbors and friends was clearly on display. There were a lot of wet eyes and emotional voices describing how they felt about us leaving. Frankly, until then, I didn't fully understand the depth of these relationships. My neighbor Steve said it would be a tough adjustment because we had been neighbors and friends for so many years. Everyone agreed, however, that this was the correct decision for us. They were all happy that we would get the support of Mike's family and the senior living facility in the future.

Members of our support network continue to assist us. Tom, my handyman, cleaned our gutters and replaced screens in the downspouts once the leaves had fallen after we left. He is going to paint the trim on the house.

When Mobility Works removed the instructor brake from my van, they were supposed to keep it and send us a refund. Instead, they put it in the van's trunk. I didn't have time to deal with that before we moved. Our neighbor, Steve, found the instructor brake in the garage, packed it up and sent it to Mobility Works, which allowed me to get a refund. Later, when I found how much Jodie liked to look through books with pictures, he went through the house and found our yearbooks. He packed them up and sent them to us. Jodie spends a significant amount of time with them now. He will periodically go through the house to turn on the faucets and flush the toilets to ensure that the traps don't dry out.* He opens the garage so our gardener, Javier, can adjust the sprinkler system when necessary.

Javier will continue to take care of the grounds and adjust the sprinkler system. Each spring he will purchase and plant flowers. I want our home and the neighborhood to continue to be attractive. Our flowers contribute to that, along with our flowering bushes and trees.

Even when we were living in our home, our neighbors, Sara and Mark, always

---

* Dried out traps can allow a sewer odor to enter the house.

alerted us to issues like sprinklers malfunctioning that they could see in our side yard that we couldn't. I know they will continue to watch for problems, as will Steve, and alert us so we can take corrective action.

Both neighbors have a key to our house. The Knox Box at our front door would allow the fire department to get quickly into the house if necessary. I expect to have the cleaning lady clean the house periodically. This continuing support allows us to know that our home will be well taken care of in our absence.

Our son and daughter-in-law had flown up to California to help us move since I wanted to take both the van and the Porsche Cayenne to Phoenix. The Porsche would serve as a backup for transportation if my van were being serviced. Also, I wanted both the wheelchair and the scooter to be taken to Phoenix in case the wheelchair was being serviced. For long trips like our move to Phoenix or a reunion, it would be more comfortable to ride in the Porsche's passenger seat than in the wheelchair in the van. When we made a stop, taking the scooter off the back of the Porsche would be much faster and more convenient than getting than wheelchair out of the van.

Lisa drove the van because she owns a Toyota Sienna. Mike drove the Porsche. Kris traveled with us and stayed a few days in Phoenix. She was a great help, making the long trip fun for Jodie and helping her transition. We were all happily surprised how well the transition went, considering how much Jodie loved our California home and our friends there. I believe the medication was a significant factor as well.

The next chapter provides information about senior care living facilities and our experiences living in one.

32

Initial Accommodations, Serious Threats

"Disasters will always come and go, leaving their victims either completely broken or steeled and seasoned and better able to face the next crop of challenges that may occur."
—Nelson Mandela, letter to Winnie Mandela, June 23, 1969,
in *Notes to the Future: Words of Wisdom* (2012)

Initial Accommodations

We were fortunate to stay in a temporary apartment in LivGenerations Ahwatukee (Liv) until the moving van arrived. We had decided to take two days for the trip. That would allow us to arrive in the early afternoon, giving us time to move in. It also had the advantage of breaking up the long trip from California to Arizona. Once we moved in, we would have access to meals in the dining room and other services. Our temporary apartment only had one bedroom but was adequate for our short-term needs. In some ways, it helped with Jodie's transition as she didn't wake up alone in a strange place. Also, I could wake her when I thought she might need to use the bathroom. While we were waiting for the moving van, we could get familiar with the facility, stock our permanent apartment with food and supplies, and meet people.

Initial Threats: Wandering and Tuberculosis Screen

Wandering

A disturbing issue arose during this period, however. Before we signed with Liv, I was asked whether Jodie wandered. Their concern was that she might walk out of the building onto a street and get into a dangerous situation. I told them that this was not an issue. Jodie had never wandered away from our house.

Shortly after we moved into the temporary apartment, someone told the Leasing Coordinator (LC) that Jodie was wandering daily and might need to go

186

into Memory Care. They advised the LC that she should talk to the family. The LC didn't talk to me; she talked to my daughter-in-law, Lisa, when she entered the facility and discussed the issue with her. She also left a voice message for our son, Mike, who did not return the call as he wanted to talk to me first.

What the Leasing Coordinator was told was greatly exaggerated, easily explained, and contained false information. When Lisa told me what happened, I was incensed! They made a trivial deal a big deal, one that threatened our ability to live there. I feared someone's motivation was to put Jodie into memory care.

I told Lisa about a couple of unusual incidents that were likely the basis for this report. While I was getting ready for breakfast one day, Jodie became angry with me and walked out of our third-floor, temporary apartment. I knew she left but decided to let her cool down. She wouldn't get on the elevator and didn't know where the steps were. She would stay on our floor and would be easy to find. One of the Assisted Living personnel saw her and came to the apartment to tell me Jodie was out in the hall. I explained that I was letting her anger with me subside and would come to get her soon. I found her immediately after that.

Later, when the movers were bringing in our belongings, there was a brief period when I was supervising the movers alone because Lisa had an appointment. I saw Jodie talking to another resident at our doorway but thought nothing of it. The next time I looked, she was no longer there. I went out into the hall where I quickly found her. She was with another resident. Jodie had knocked on her door looking for me.

At that point, no one knew us. The lady intended to walk her to the front desk. That incident wouldn't have happened if I had not been supervising the movers alone for a short period. I am always with her. But in that situation, the movers had to keep the door open and I had been momentarily distracted. Once the residents knew us, they would have called me or brought Jodie to our apartment. There was no chance Jodie would have gone outside without me and certainly not in cold weather, which was the case then. She gets cold easily. I have great difficulty getting her to go outside with me in cold or hot weather, even to go to medical appointments.

Lisa immediately went to see the LC and the Liv personnel who had raised the issue and encouraged the LC to contact our family. Knowing the facts, Lisa asked them to tell the LC how many times Jodie's wandering had happened. The LC quickly realized the issue had been exaggerated.

Then I met with the LC. I started by telling her that I was upset that she hadn't come to me first. I told her that I was the principal, the decision-maker, and the one with the facts. I made it clear to her that moving Jodie to Memory Care would destroy both Jodie and me. That was not going to happen until, and unless, I decided it was time for that. If that were their intention, we would move out that night. The LC became emotional and apologized for not talking to me first. She said had she done so, she would have understood that this was a trivial matter and would have told everyone to "chill." We previously had a great relationship with her and maintained that.

Nevertheless, I realized that Liv created a much different situation than our home regarding wandering. It is easy for Jodie to walk out of the apartment door but still be in the building, unlike our home. She won't go outside; nothing dangerous will happen. However, there was a much higher potential for wandering in Liv. I needed to deal with it.

My concern about Jodie perhaps wandering at Liv was realized after we moved into our permanent apartment. I set up a blockade in front of the door each night with a fan and trash cans. That solved the problem for some time. But early one morning, she removed the blockade and slipped out while I was sleeping. When I realized she was gone, I turned the wheelchair to maximum speed and quickly found her. Later, while I was in the bathroom, she left again. I again found her down the hall.

Subsequently, there was a night where I couldn't sleep. That afternoon, I took a nap. I had removed the blockade that morning and forgot to rebuild it. Jodie got out and knocked on someone's apartment door. She came back to our room with that resident and opened the door. However, the lady who was with her, apparently thinking this wasn't Jodie's apartment, insisted that she come out into the hallway. I heard the conversation and brought her back, but it was clear that I needed a better solution.

The solution I found was the GE Personal Security Window/Door Alarm shown to the right. It costs less than $10 on Amazon and comes in a 2-pack. It takes only a few minutes to install it with the adhesive supplied. It can be set either to chime once when the door is opened, or to sound a loud alarm while the door is open. It is a proximity sensor.

The alarm is very loud and stops Jodie immediately. She then quickly shuts the door. Problem solved.

It gives me peace of mind when I am sleeping, using the bathroom, or showering. In those situations, I activate the alarm. Hopefully, she never realizes how to turn it off. It is designed so that it isn't obvious how to do that. The device is small, and the switch that sets or turns off the device is tiny. In the picture to the right, you can see it on the side of the device. Because it is barely visible from a front view, I took the picture at an angle.

After many months the alarm has been 100 percent effective.

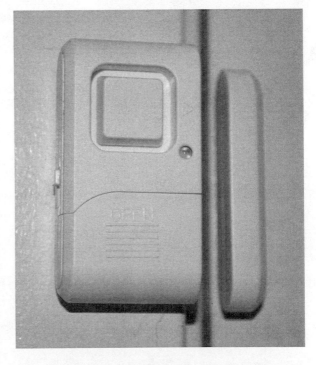

Door alarm (photograph by the author).

Tuberculosis Screen

If you live in a senior living facility in Arizona, you must get a tuberculosis screen every year. Generally, this is done with a small injection in the underside of your arm. A week later, the arm is examined to see whether there is a positive reaction. I knew this was not going to happen with Jodie because she won't take shots or allow blood draws, a huge worry. What would we do if we had to leave because of this?

About a month after we moved in, Jodie got a very severe headache. I called a mobile urgent care organization. They examined her and said she might be having a stroke and should go to the emergency room immediately. I didn't see any symptoms to suggest that was the case, but we went anyway. The hospital found nothing serious. They suggested the headache might have been caused by dehydration. Earlier, I had learned that a chest X-ray would suffice for a TB screen. I took advantage of us being at a hospital and asked them to give Jodie the X-ray.

It was challenging to get Jodie to cooperate. I had to accompany and continually urge her to allow the technicians to do what was needed. The hospital personnel were very accommodating. To get the X-ray, they relaxed requirements, allowing her to wear some clothing they would normally remove and taking fewer images than usual. It was a great relief to know the tuberculous screening for this year was now no longer a problem.

The next chapter explains the process of our social integration.

33

Social Integration

"Success is not final, failure is not fatal, it is the courage to continue that counts."

—Winston Churchill

Initially, we found it difficult to make friends or learn much about other people in the facility. We were new, whereas other residents had established relationships. All we would get was a nod or hello, no real communication. At first, we thought that many of the advertised features were not as satisfactory as hoped. Some lectures were canceled because of a lack of interest. Movies were played in the theater, but few, if any, people were there. Bingo is well attended, but we are not interested in bingo and it didn't seem very useful for creating relationships. Everyone was intent on studying their bingo boards. Katie, one of our granddaughters, arranged to have tea in the tea room with Jodie but no one showed up.

My opinion about social activities changed later. For example, we learned later that teas are usually well attended but there was a conflicting event the day Katie came for tea. We attended music shows performed in the lobby or the ballroom. When we attended wine-tasting parties it was more productive, and we started to meet people. Later, because of COVID restrictions, Liv arranged a Mother's Day parade that made the papers. They also created many virtual activities that will outlive the COVID period. It is also true that the many hours a day I spent writing this book caused me to avoid taking advantage of some of the social opportunities.

We soon realized that the best way to meet people was to join them at meals. As a result, we were meeting many people in a short period. It was embarrassing to have people address us by name and not only not know their names, or even whether we had met them. Due to my life-long inability to remember names, I created a LivGenerations Residents document. Over time, I was able to include:

1. Names
2. Apartment numbers
3. Physical description
4. Mobility equipment description where appropriate
5. Residents' council members and their responsibilities
6. How we met them

7. Who their friends were
8. Clubs they joined and
9. Information about their career and families

Before I went to the restaurant, I would look through the document to jog my memory.

It didn't take long before I was well known in the facility because I started sending informational flyers to all the residents. I had observed that many of the people at Liv use improperly sized walkers. As a result, many people walked bent over with the walker too far out in front of them. This would not protect them from falling and can create back problems.

I approached Liv and suggested that they do something about it. They agreed it was a problem but thought they had done enough about it. I offered to meet with people who might be interested in learning more about the proper use and sizing of walkers and sent some information about this subject to the activities person at Liv, but there was no reaction.

I decided to do something about it myself, so I published "How to Size and Use a Walker," a one-page document (flyer) wherein I provided information regarding proper sizing and best use of a walker. It contained my name, apartment number and cell phone number. I used material from this book to create it. I offered to talk with anyone who wanted to learn more. Liv copied it and Jodie and I delivered it on all three floors. I received some positive comments from the residents about it. One told me she was going to resize her walker based on information in the flyer. Others ignored it and are still using improperly sized walkers.

Deciding that this was a helpful thing to the residents, I published "Preparing for Emergencies" focused on Smart911, also taken from this book. It was very well received. Multiple people told me that they, and others they knew, were going to sign up. Some said to me that they appreciated what I was doing. A member of the resident's council asked whether I would be interested in becoming a member. I declined for two reasons. I was very busy with caregiving and writing this book. More importantly, Jodie would have to come with me and would be a disruption. More people now stopped to talk to us at that point.

More flyers followed, all taken from the book *Improve Your Odds of Getting Insurance Coverage for Medical Equipment*, providing a procedure explaining how to utilize, prepare and coordinate your doctor, occupational therapist, and equipment supplier to improve your odds of success. It also included a list of Medicare codes that would work.

I expected to stop producing flyers at that point, but that changed at one of the wine tastings. We sat with a group of people, one of whom is about 90. He has macular degeneration, which is causing him to go blind. He seemed depressed and pointed a finger to his head, suggesting suicide. I didn't take that seriously, but it confirmed my impression that he suffered from depression. When seeing him make that motion, a woman in the group said: "No, don't do that."

I decided to make a joke about it to lighten the mood and said: "I think I just saw Bob [one of his friends sitting at the table] reaching for his gun." The guy started laughing. I spent some time talking to him. I told him he didn't have to give up on doing the everyday things in life. He could get a dog and other assistance. I mentioned the essay "Attitude" by Charles R. Swindoll and explained its message. As I left the table, he told me he enjoyed talking to me; I had given him hope.

I made a copy of "Attitude" and gave it to his friend Bob to read to him. Bob strongly encouraged me to send out a flyer about that as well. That led to a flyer titled "Attitude." Again, several people made favorable comments about the flyer.

Jodie and I were eating with an older couple one evening. The woman mentioned that she had trouble reaching things. I asked whether she had a reacher, also known as a grabber, and found she did not. I own two myself. I keep one at each of the two places where I spend most of my time, my bed and my lift chair, so I did not have a spare. I decided to buy two additional reachers and gave one to her. I mentioned to a few people that I had an extra reacher and was willing to acquire more.

A few weeks later, I learned that two residents had bad falls. One fell while reaching for something and broke her hip. I wasn't sure of the cause of the second resident's fall but knew some falls could be avoided by using reachers. Another resident asked for the extra reacher. That led me to publish "Reacher/Grabber for Convenience and Safety," wherein I offered to purchase one for anyone who needed one. Only two asked for one. They both insisted on paying for them. This flyer was well-received by the community. I even got very favorable comments about that flyer on several occasions from the Executive Director of Liv.

Much later, I was reminded of the obvious. You can provide excellent advice but it does no good if the advice is ignored. A caregiver came to my apartment and asked for my phone number for another resident. When the resident called me, I discovered that she was the lady that had fallen and broken her hip; the very reason that I wrote the flyer on reachers. She wanted me to come to her apartment to help her adjust the size of her new walker. I learned that she had trouble getting Medicare approval so her son bought one on Amazon. It was too tall for her; even at its lowest setting, the handles were too high.

I assume she never read the flyer on the procedure for getting Medicare approval because it would have been easy to obtain approval. The result was that she paid for an incorrectly sized walker. How she knew to contact me is unknown. Possibly the resident next door to her, who is on the residents' council, told her to contact me.

I have been encouraged to write more flyers by residents. I will only write another if I see a need or someone asks me a question for which I have useful information that might be of interest to others as well.

Another factor for not writing more flyers is that we are mostly confined to our apartments due to COVID-19. To leave briefly to walk in the community or walk outside on the facilities grounds, we must wear masks. Jodie won't do that. So at this time, it would not be possible to deliver a flyer if I were to write one. Other impacts of the virus are discussed in Chapter 35.

One of the unexpected positive effects of living in a senior living facility was the effect on Jodie's social life, the subject of the next chapter.

34

Jodie's Successful Adaptation, Unexpected Positives

"Success is sweet, the sweeter if long delayed and attained through manifold struggles and defeats."
—A. Bronson Alcott, in *Table-Talk* (1877)

We moved into Liv in the middle of November 2019. In the first weeks of living in LivGenerations, there were some challenging times. At one point, I thought I couldn't manage the situation much longer. However, by December, everything was going very well. Jodie's condition was even better than in California before the crisis that led to our relocation. One indication of her positive adaptation to Liv is that she does not spend much time with her "dogs" anymore.

But there are many more important indications. She doesn't throw things. She doesn't put her fingers in her mouth and pretend to bite them. She used to do that when she was angry but she is rarely angry now.

Her bathroom issues have almost completely disappeared. She doesn't put extra toilet paper everywhere, in part because I don't provide more than one roll at a time and it is always on the dispenser. She often gets up on her own and goes to the bathroom in the middle of the night.

There is no violence.

I believe there are many reasons for her substantial improvement. They are listed below:

1. We found the right medication and the correct dosage.
2. She is thrilled with our apartment and the view we have from it.
3. She constantly tells me how much she likes it here when we are in the dining room or walk outside.
4. Our family's social life blossomed, something we didn't have in California. We go out to dinner with our son's family and sometimes eat together at Liv. Lisa (our daughter-in-law) appreciates getting a break from making dinner. My son and I watch sporting events like Penn State football and the Super Bowl. Lisa has free time during the day so we go to movies and have lunch afterward.
5. Much to my surprise, Jodie's social life at Liv is better than it was in

California. We don't have the close relationships we had in California. However, at best, we saw our friends in California once a week. Here there are multiple opportunities every week to socialize with people. We sit with people at lunch and dinner. Every Wednesday, there is a wine tasting that encourages conversations with new people. There are other chances to socialize as well.

6. These frequent social interactions are incredibly valuable for Jodie. Her true nature is on display for everyone to see. They recognize that she has a good heart. Jodie has always been kind to people and wants to help them. Often she tries to give people her food. I'm not entirely sure why, but this has become a prominent feature of her personality in Liv. People recognize that she's not always able to convey in words what she wants to say but realize that she is a lovely person. She compliments residents and the restaurant's servers on their looks, clothing, hair, and accessories. She tells them how nice they are, that they have been very kind to her, and that she loves them. Because Jodie is so kind to them, they, in return, are kind to her. This constant feedback is an essential reason for her happiness at Liv.

7. She has little memory of her California friends and our old home.

8. There is less stress and more time to enjoy life because we don't have to cook, wash dishes, clean the apartment, or make beds.

9. Jodie was not eating enough in California, and the variety of the food she would eat was limited. She eats more here. I always order for her and choose a greater variety of food than she used to eat. Better nutrition may be a factor in her happiness.

10. Probably the most significant factor is that I have taken more of a laissez-faire approach to caregiving. For example, getting Jodie dressed was always stressful. Near the end of our time in California, she would sometimes wear the same clothes to bed that she wore during the day. Preventing that was challenging, stressful, and usually impossible. Since we moved to Liv, I stopped trying to get her to change her clothing. As a result, battles that would have accomplished nothing have been avoided.

Not having to get Jodie dressed in the morning is an excellent time-saver and stress avoider. Now she wears the same clothing 24 hours a day for two or more days. When she is cold, she puts on a warmer top which changes the look. Her slacks get changed when she gets them wet.

The frequency of bathroom issues is very low now as she has gotten more familiar with the apartment and her anxiety has declined. She refuses to wear incontinence underwear. After many futile attempts to change this, I had to accept it. In any case, the need for them is significantly lower now.

Brushing her teeth is another problem. In the first three months here, I think she has brushed her teeth only once or twice, although she brushed several times a day in California. I suggest that she brush her teeth and put the toothbrush and toothpaste near her. When she won't do it, I drop the subject.

My research indicated that being more flexible is desirable, but I found that it was not just desirable, but necessary for her happiness and my sanity. The result of these changes is a much happier environment, an essential objective of caregiving.

Some readers will probably think this laissez-faire approach is terrible. But they are not in my shoes and don't fully understand the fruitlessness of repeatedly attempting that which cannot be accomplished and the negative atmosphere trying creates. My advice to caregivers is to be unconcerned about what others think. Each situation is different and requires an approach that will be successful in that situation. Always remember what your objective is. My belief is it is to create a loving, happy life, not only for the person you are caring for but also for yourself. If you are overstressed and unhappy, your patient will also be. This is not healthy for either of you.

I don't mean to imply that Jodie's behavior in social situations is always great. After a few weeks of positivity, one day a new resident joined us for dinner. Jodie was displaying Sundowner Syndrome before dinner. She became agitated and kept saying we had to go back to our apartment. (I don't know why, but this happens every time we leave the apartment, even to go to our son's home.)

This time she repeatedly left the table and walked away. She would not eat any of her food. The woman who joined us thought she had caused the problem. I assured her that she hadn't, but she offered to leave. I told her if she felt more comfortable leaving, she should. I explained that the cause was Sundowner Syndrome and explained what it was. She decided to stay. When Jodie came back again, the woman asked her how she was feeling. Jodie "threw her a look," said nothing, and left permanently. I had to apologize, and without finishing my meal, leave the new resident sitting alone at the table.

As a young parent, I learned that people who don't know you or what you are dealing with make quick judgments about your capabilities. I couldn't be prouder of our son, Mike. He is a great son, brother, husband, and father. He is highly respected and successful in his career. But, when he was young, he was quite a challenge for us at times. We would get disapproving looks from strangers, judging us, indicating they thought we weren't good parents. It didn't affect me. I knew they had no idea how well Jodie and I were parenting. I just thought less of them.

Some of the comments the woman made before we left reminded me of those long-ago experiences. I sensed that this resident, who had met us for just a few minutes, concluded that I couldn't care for Jodie properly, and memory care might be in order. I have learned not to get upset with other people's opinions. This applies to how people might react to how Jodie dresses, my care, or anything else. I am the only one who intimately knows what I am dealing with, and I am confident that I am doing the best job possible; no one else would do as well. My objective is to make sure Jodie is happy, feels loved, and is safe. So far, I am certain that this has been accomplished.

In retrospect, I decided that I should take a different approach when we are conversing with others. In this case, the resident was on my left and Jodie was on my right. When I was talking to her, Jodie was behind me. Typically, we are alone or with just one other couple. With four people at the table, my gaze would move from person to person. It would also be more likely that someone else would engage Jodie when I was otherwise engaged. I had not met this woman before and spent time talking to her to learn more about her. Jodie possibly felt ignored.

I believe the primary cause was Sundowners, but my inattention could have been a contributing factor that I now needed to address. Jodie currently has difficulty making relevant contributions to discussions in social situations, but I resolved to engage her in the conversation. Initial results have been reasonably effective, but I need to work on this continually. When involved, she is happy making many comments, a great deal of which aren't understood or relevant, but that doesn't matter. Most people smile and nod in agreement or say yes.

We had a breakthrough in late January 2020. I have detailed the large number of routine things that Jodie doesn't do anymore. An important one is that she has not taken a shower for over two years and does not wash her hair. There is a salon in Liv. I decided to get a haircut there and took Jodie along to see how they might wash her hair.

We were fortunate in that the appointment after mine had been canceled. The hairdresser and I encouraged Jodie to have her hair washed. I knew it was worth a try but didn't think we would succeed. Surprisingly, it seemed like she might reluctantly cooperate. In the beginning, it looked like Jodie was going to get up and leave. After much encouragement, she stayed. She was grimacing and clearly unhappy but allowed the hairdresser to wash and dry her hair. When she saw how nice her hair looked, she was delighted. That allowed us to get her hair cut a little shorter. As I talked with the hairdresser, I learned that she cares for troubled children. If they go down on the floor, she goes down with them to get the job done. She was well qualified to help Jodie.

Jodie's hair looked so much better, and she received multiple compliments. I had primed some people to give her compliments, but many were unsolicited. This breakthrough was possible only because of the environment in which we now live, enhanced by the fact that she's happy here and is on a higher Celexa dose. I'm hoping that we may be able to continue doing this. Because of closures due to COVID-19, I am concerned that that happy experience will have been so long ago that she is not likely to remember how well it went. That hairdresser no longer comes to Liv, which reduces Jodie's chances of getting her hair done again.

One of my challenges is that I have to be with Jodie at all times. I cannot do anything or go anywhere without her. This situation has definite negative social implications. As mentioned earlier, I have been asked whether I would be interested in being a member of the Residents' Council. I was also asked by a few people to join the bridge club. It would be a much-needed outlet if I would join them, but my reply is that I don't believe either is possible, as Jodie has to be with me and she might be disruptive. My need to concentrate on finishing this book would be a deterrent as well, but I would find the time if it were not for the other concern.

In the next chapter, I will discuss Jodie's medical condition and more information on COVID-19 effects.

35

Final Update and Closing

*"However difficult life may seem, there is always something you can
do and succeed at."*

—Stephen Hawking

My friend and fellow author, Bill Huber, once said to me, "Writing never ends. At some point, you just have to stop." This is an excellent place to follow that advice. This chapter represents the end of our journey as far as this book is concerned. To close, I will update Jodie's medical condition and describe the effects COVID-19 has had on us while living in LivGenerations Ahwatukee.

Medical Power of Attorney,
Achieved Through Perseverance!

In Chapter 29: The Crisis: Big Problems, Out of Answers, I mentioned that I needed to get a medical power of attorney to care for Jodie properly but had not been able to get one. While we were at the hospital dealing with Jodie's headaches and getting the TB scan, I talked to a social worker about getting a medical power of attorney. She provided the appropriate form.

Considering both Jodie's condition and my own, I prepared one for each of us. We signed them at our son's home in front of one of Lisa's friends, an unrelated witness. To complete the process, I needed a letter from a doctor confirming that Jodie could not make rational, independent decisions regarding healthcare, finances, and legal matters. Jodie's psychiatrist provided what we needed. At that point, we finally had both the right medication and the ability to execute medical and other decisions.

Under the doctor's orders, I gradually increased Jodie's medication dosage. By January 2020, her situation improved significantly, but some issues remain. She still has anxieties related to having her nails cut, taking showers, and going to doctors or dentists. She no longer brushes her teeth. She is afraid of the cars on the road when she is in the van. The doctor tried lowering the dose of the anti-anxiety medication and adding an anti-psychotic drug. The result was disturbing, so we dropped the anti-psychotic and returned to the higher dose of anti-anxiety medication. I have no answer for those behaviors and may never have one. Otherwise, things are excellent now.

COVID-19 Pandemic Affects Life at Liv

Our nephew, Brian Reed, sounded the alarm regarding COVID-19 for our extended family very early. Many of his predictions came true, including panic buying that would empty store shelves. He was most worried about my generation. He recommended that Jodie and I move out of Liv to our son's house. Making the modifications to Mike's home to make that work would have been challenging; showering would have been impossible. But those aren't the reasons we didn't do it. There were five other people in Mike's house, all of whom were interacting with other people. Moving there seemed to create more risk than sheltering in our apartment at Liv.

While Liv complied with federal and state guidelines, I was not sure they were sufficient for us. Jodie is 81; I am 79 and have asthma, a precondition. I created ways for us to avoid social interaction until the precautions were more stringent. We didn't attend any group activities. When we still had dining room service, we would sit alone at a table. We stayed mostly in the apartment. Our daughter-in-law, Lisa, bought wipes that I used on door handles and other surfaces we had to touch when we left the apartment. But, through a series of steps, Liv made the changes we needed.

Group Activities Were Canceled

Informal groups of up to 10 could get together but, due to initial non-compliance regarding social distancing, they placed "X" marks (later stickers) on the pavement in the courtyard and the ballroom showing where people could sit. We still didn't join them. Later, everyone had to wear masks if they weren't in their apartments. The maximum group size was later reduced to six.

The Dining Room Was Closed

All meals were delivered. It was not possible to deliver that many meals hot, so often they were just warm. You didn't know exactly when the meal was coming. If you couldn't immediately eat because you were in the middle of something, the food was cold. These problems were unavoidable and one of the many effects of the virus.

Servers weren't supposed to enter the apartment but occasionally did to assist us. Assisted living personnel have to be able to enter apartments where that service is provided. Given our situation, an assisted living employee would often accompany the servers and bring the food into our apartment.

Among the significant advantages of living in a senior living facility is that you have many meal choices, don't have to make meals, set the table or clean up afterward. Delivered meals eliminated all of these advantages except making the meals, thus significantly increasing my workload. I now had to clean and dispose of containers and wash glasses, silverware, and plates.

As Jodie is a finicky eater, and I need gluten-free (GF) food, a high percentage of the delivered meals initially went down the disposal. Liv had never seemed very concerned about providing many GF choices. When we ate in the dining room there were more choices. While I was unhappy about the limited GF choices, the problem was less significant because I could always choose a hamburger, hot dog or other "always available" items. It became more significant when meals were delivered. I started to use DoorDash occasionally as a result.

For weeks, they would sometimes deliver food that wasn't GF. Sometimes they told me something was gluten-free, but I was suspicious and checked to find out that it wasn't. The dining room got calls from me for many meals. I asked them to mark all items "GF" if they were GF. Most of the time they did, but I often had to call the restaurant or chase down the hall after the servers to get clarification. Even after the improvements mentioned below, I occasionally still got unmarked containers containing food that was not gluten-free.

There was a dramatic improvement in delivering GF food near the end of April. Many more GF options were provided. More soups were GF for everyone. When GF soups were available, they would give me extra soup that I could keep in the refrigerator, thus enabling me to have soup on days when the soup wasn't GF. Some meals were modified for me to be GF, for example, by not putting gravy on the potatoes.

If none of the options were GF and couldn't be easily modified, they made a special meal using one of the suggestions I provided for those situations. They bought GF bread and delivered a loaf to me. They started making sandwiches using GF bread. After not having any dessert for a long time, they started giving me ice cream for dessert. The epidemic indirectly led to an improvement in GF options that hopefully will last after we return to eating in the dining room.

I believe there were several reasons for the dramatic shift in GF food availability. Proactively, I often called the kitchen with questions and reasonable complaints. Also, I had developed positive relationships with the Director of Dining Room Services and a couple of chefs.

Two more reasons are our relationships with the servers and my relationship with the Executive Director (ED) of the facility. The servers love Jodie and are very interested in my book. Several of the servers occasionally lingered after they delivered the food to ask about the book. They wanted to know what it was about, why I was writing it, and the progress I was making.

I mentioned earlier that the Executive Director was positively affected by the flyer that I wrote on reachers. Later, I was having difficulty getting the information I wanted on the cost and content of assisted living and memory care for this book. I asked to meet with him about this. To help him understand what my book was about, I sent some passages to him before our meeting. I didn't expect him to read them in advance, but I saw that he had highlighted many of them when I entered his office. He told me he was moved by what he read and that he wanted to help. He promised to get the information I requested and did so in a follow-up meeting. The big surprise was that he also offered to introduce me to a potential Foreword writer he knew.

During our first meeting, I had told him we were very happy living in Liv and felt safe during the virus pandemic. I mentioned in passing that one of the challenges I still faced was the limited gluten-free food choices available. That might have been one of the causes of the expansion of GF choices.

Getting Outside and Interacting

In some ways, it is fortunate that the pandemic hit at this time of the year for those living in Arizona. Some of the best days to be outside in Arizona are in late March and early April. There are many weeks of the year when one would not want to spend much time outside because of the high temperatures. Before the pandemic impacted us, the weather was very pleasant, and we walked down the street every day after lunch.

Pandemic-related restrictions effectively quarantined us in our apartment and confined us to Liv's grounds. At least there remained the opportunity to enjoy the grounds around Liv and the internal courtyard. We continued to take walks around the buildings and through the grounds.

Others took advantage of opportunities that we avoided because of the virus, our age, and my asthma. Many people formed small groups in the courtyard, which would become impossible during the hottest part of the year. There was considerable time for discussion. For many residents, this was an excellent opportunity to build stronger relationships. As relatively new residents, this would have been very helpful for us, but we didn't join them. Jodie is very social and has no understanding of the need for social distancing and not touching things. I always avoided walking near people because she might violate the prohibitions. Compounding the problem, while no one had been diagnosed with COVID-19, not all residents were rigorous about social distancing. On a couple of occasions, someone reached out and shook Jodie's hand. I always carried disinfectant wipes, but Jodie wouldn't let me wipe her hands, and forcing it would have caused a scene.

As the temperature rose in May, we started walking in the early morning. The flowering bushes and trees are beautiful; the exercise is good for Jodie; we get vitamin D from the sun and enjoy the breeze.

Then Liv instituted more extreme steps consistent with the President's Corona Virus Task Force, including confinement and face masks.

Confinement and Facemasks

If we left Liv's grounds for any reason, we would be quarantined in our apartments for two weeks. It was also against the rules to meet with friends or relatives on the grounds. Some relatives drove their cars to the side or back of the building and walked up to the patios to deliver items. At times, the visitors set up a chair outside the porch to talk with their relatives. Some residents left the premises in their cars or were picked up by a relative. Those actions resulted in quarantines when management discovered that they had occurred. At least two people decided to move out of Liv because of these restrictions. Another kept the apartment but moved to a second home they have in the mountains. Later they left Liv permanently.

We could not visit with our family. All deliveries had to be received outside the building and sanitized before they were delivered. We could not enter any part of the building other than our apartment without wearing masks. We were also supposed to wear masks if anyone came into the apartment. We were to wear masks and meet Liv personnel at the door for our food, mail or any other reason.

Unfortunately, Jodie was unwilling to wear a mask. We followed the rules for weeks, but since Jodie wouldn't wear a mask, we were effectively quarantined in our apartment. It was having a negative impact on both our mental health and Jodie's physical health. I finally decided to ignore the mask rule for Jodie so we could walk outside but carefully continued social distancing.

To avoid any interaction with residents, we left through a side door that was very close to our apartment. We then had to reenter through the main entrance to the reception area. The risk was that they would quarantine us, but we were effectively doing that already. After entering the building, a short walk would take us to an entrance to the courtyard. Most of the time, few, if any, residents were in the courtyard due to the increasingly high temperature in Arizona at that time. At the end of the courtyard, a door opened right next to our apartment. This procedure avoided almost all interaction with other residents.

A second meeting with the ED occurred when we had to wear masks. I told him that we'd have to do it by phone, or he would have to exempt Jodie from having to wear a mask. He allowed her to come to the meeting without a mask.

I have not had trouble with any member of the staff regarding her lack of a mask. Everyone knows I have done everything I can to get her to wear it. It just isn't possible. They love Jodie and several have told me they are impressed with how well I am dealing with her. Those factors probably account for this acceptance.

The confinement directive significantly impacted medical and dental appointments. We had to cancel medical appointments. I had just had a temporary crown put in place by my dentist and had an appointment to install the permanent crown. I planned to reschedule that appointment anyway because I was disturbed that everyone in the dentist's office wanted to shake my hand. For a medical institution, that made no sense to me and I told them so. They changed their policy, but I postponed the crown's replacement until the confinement rules at Liv were relaxed.

There were two other significant medical impacts. I was being treated with medication for an eye problem caused by a virus that affected my retina and significantly degraded vision in my right eye. At my last appointment, the doctor told me to reduce the medication levels. I complied, but my vision started to degrade. When I was able to talk to the doctor, he had me return to the previous levels, which improved the situation. The downside is that long-term use of the medication can have negative consequences, and it was uncertain when I could see him again.

The other medical issue was that we needed a new GP when we moved to Arizona. We found a well-respected one but we had to wait for months to see her. After waiting for a few months, the doctor canceled it because of the virus when the appointment was coming up. We had to reschedule it as a new patient, which delayed the appointment for additional months.

Celebration During the Pandemic

May 10, 2020, was Mother's Day. To commemorate that, Liv organized a wonderful Mother's Day Parade. Fifty decorated vehicles drove around the facility blowing their horns, shouting good wishes and waving to us. Everyone thoroughly enjoyed it. Below is a picture of our son and daughter-in-law's white Toyota van, showing our grandkids, from left to right, Lindsey, Zach, and Katie as they were preparing to enter the parade.

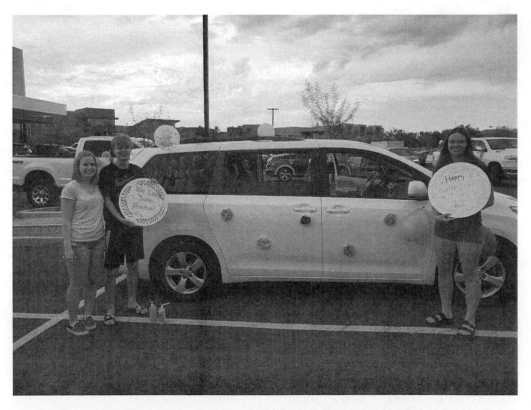

Van and grandkids (left to right) Lindsey Reed, Zach Reed and Katie Reed at Mother's Day Parade (photograph by Lisa Reed).

Conclusion

In the Appendices, I cover four topics that everyone should consider as they age:

1. Senior living facilities that may be available in your area
2. The pros and cons of long-term care insurance
3. Preparation of documents your heirs will need in case of your death
4. How to provide ready access to the documents your heirs will need

While this is the last chapter of the book, our journey is far from over. Life here in Liv has been better than I expected. The support we get from our family is terrific. When COVID-19 recedes, life will be even better when we can resume spending time with our family again and all activities resume at Liv.

While I was writing this chapter, Liv notified us of some scheduled relaxations in the rules including, seeing relatives briefly, going to medical appointments, opening the salon and increasing the dining choices. Other changes are planned for the future so our quality of life will gradually improve until we return to normal.

As Jodie and I both have untreatable, progressive diseases, I know there is an uncertain and troubling future for us. That is the case for anyone with a progressive illness or any illness that has no treatment. But with a positive attitude, perseverance, love, and ingenuity, we have achieved a lifetime of happiness and have overcome or mitigated the challenges thrown at us. You can too!

I sincerely hope you find the information in this book enhances your life and your ability to overcome the challenges you will face.

Epilogue

"Everything can be taken from a man but one thing: the last of the human freedoms—to choose one's attitude in any given set of circumstances, to choose one's own way."
—Viktor Frankl, in *Man's Search for Meaning* (1946)

When I finished writing this book in June 2020, Jodie and I were doing very well. It was the perfect way to finish the book because our situation demonstrated the book's basic premise that one could overcome severe challenges and continue to live a happy, fulfilling life.

The very next month we experienced a series of disasters that began with me breaking my leg. As I was getting up from bed at about 3 a.m. to check on Jodie, I must have stepped on a shoe during my transfer to the wheelchair. This caused me to fall. The bone above my knee snapped in two, making a trip to the hospital necessary. All I could think about during the ride to the hospital was how to take care of Jodie. I knew my son's family was in Mexico. I called my son's mother-in-law and the homecare company that I had previously engaged for just this type of emergency. If you are a caregiver, having a backup plan like this is an important precaution.

Shortly after that, LivGenerations Ahwatukee (Liv) convinced me to move Jodie to Memory Care while I was in the hospital. They said that she would get better care at a much lower cost in Memory Care. That was the worst decision of my life and led to devastating results!

Being alone without your spouse and caregiver is traumatic for anyone, particularly for someone with Alzheimer's. Removing Jodie from the familiar surroundings of her apartment, bed and bathroom compounded the problem. I was told she adapted well but later learned that was untrue. She didn't go to bed for two nights and was wandering around looking for me. As traumatic as that was, other life-changing events followed.

Jodie rarely fell before, but she had two severe falls in less than a week. First, she fell and broke her wrist. After getting a brace on her wrist, she was returned to Memory Care, where she fell again, this time breaking her hip. In addition to hip/leg surgery, surgery was required for her wrist to install a plate and screws as she was no longer weight-bearing.

A hip fracture can be a death sentence for someone over 80. An Alzheimer's patient suffering that kind of trauma generally suffers a precipitate decline in cognition. That happened to Jodie and resulted in life-altering consequences for both of us. I understand that she was given Ativan while in the Memory Care Unit to make it less difficult to shower her. Ativan is a drug I had never used. I got it for emergency use only, not for showers; they knew that. The hard lesson here is that when you turn caregiving over to others, you need to be very specific in writing about the medications they can use and for what purpose.

I now know what the effects of Ativan are on Jodie. After we had returned to our apartment, I gave it to her so she could tolerate the first Covid-19 vaccine. For the first four hours after taking this drug, she was completely asleep and did not react as she got the vaccine. For the next four hours, she woke up briefly from time to time but immediately went back to sleep. It was evident that you had to watch her constantly for hours after giving her Ativan. Otherwise, she could fall, possibly breaking a bone. She is 82 years old and has osteoporosis. When I gave Ativan to her, we had 24/7 care so there was no risk of a fall. It is impossible to get that kind of care in Memory Care or Assisted Living where their caregivers have several patients under their care.

Jodie experienced all this trauma in a new environment without our family or me to comfort her. I was in the hospital; Covid-19 visiting restrictions kept our family away.

I realized that it was critical to get Jodie assigned to my rehab hospital. I feared I would lose her in fundamental ways unless I could be with her to help. After fighting the bureaucracy, I succeeded in having her transferred to the hospital where I was but was distressed to see her condition when she arrived. I helped get her to eat and drink more and participate in physical and occupational therapy.

When we were discharged from the rehab hospital, we could not return to our apartment due to our physical conditions and the need for daily medication. We then stayed in what they call Signature Care at Liv, which is a version of Assisted Living. I had several concerns while living there. The most important issue was Jodie's safety. Fortunately, she could walk, which I was told was unexpected. However, state law for this type of facility meant that we could not restrain her from falling out of bed or getting out of bed and then falling. Jodie surprised us one morning when we saw she was not in bed. She was sitting on the toilet in the bathroom. I couldn't get the manager in charge to agree to have the caregivers check on Jodie as frequently as I thought was necessary. Even what she did agree to was often disregarded. Eventually, I hired external caregivers to stay with us at night to protect Jodie.

Another issue was pain management. Jodie was in so much pain at night that she would plead with God and me to help her. She couldn't stand it! It is soul-crushing to lie in bed and hear this agony from your wife and not be able to do anything to help. It was happening every night for hours,* and it didn't help

---

* Alzheimers patients may feel pain more acutely. See https://www.webmd.com/alzheimers/news/20060922/pain-problem-in-alzheimers-disease.

that the medicine wasn't always delivered on time and there was frequent confusion over what and when she was to get it. The management of that portion of the facility later changed.

Jodie felt like she was being tortured because of the shots she was getting to avoid blood clots, the Tylenol suppositories she was given several times a day, cold showers, and being roughly handed at times. It caused her to fight back. (This carried over to some degree after we returned to our apartment but was solved mainly with good caregivers and astute caregiving techniques that evolved as her condition changed.)

I knew it was vital to get us back to our apartment as soon as possible. To accomplish this, I had to be able to function myself without help. I was able to regain all the capabilities I had before the fall but had to make adjustments to some of my equipment. With Jodie's diminished capabilities, it would now be necessary to have 24/7 caregivers because I could no longer care for her by myself. I had to find a way to dispense her medication because the caregivers were prohibited from giving medication.

We were able to get back into our apartment, where Jodie was much more comfortable and where we could live together as we had before. The dispensing of medication solution was liquid Tylenol. Jodie would not swallow pills and I couldn't give her a suppository, but I could make a drink she liked that included liquid Tylenol.

I found a company that could provide good caregivers around the clock. While we have had a significant turnover of caregivers, on balance, this has worked out well. There was an unexpected benefit to having these caregivers. They all fall in love with Jodie and she feels this love from multiple people.

So many things have changed since I finished this book that it is impossible to list them all. The majority of these changes are positive developments. For example:

- Her paranoia is gone.
- She is now being cared for by Hospice of the Valley, an outstanding organization.
- We are visited once a week by Jodie's nurse.
- Two ladies come twice a week to give her showers.
- A social worker comes about every two weeks.
- A nurse practitioner is available by phone for consultations and comes every two months to ensure that Jodie still qualifies for hospice.
- All incontinency-related items and drugs are provided on the same day when necessary.
- Her fingernails and toenails are cut.
- A chaplain comes periodically.
- She has received both doses of the COVID-19 vaccine.

One of my primary responsibilities is to plan for our uncertain future. For example, before I finished this Epilogue, I learned that I have Melanoma but currently don't know how serious it is. I always plan for the worst case. The experience of older adults who have been married for many years is that when one dies, the other soon follows. Given our close, loving relationship, I suspect Jodie would not survive long if I died first. It is vital for me to ensure she will have the best possible life if I predecease her. I am doing everything I can to survive her but have little control over that. I requested that my family not put Jodie in Memory Care in the event of my death. I want her under the care of Hospice of the Valley and placed in a group home that they recommend.

We continue to enjoy a very happy life. This is primarily possible because of our very strong, loving relationship and ability to afford the necessary care. I am well aware that less happy times will come. The most important thing is to enjoy life as best you can as long as you can. We are certainly doing that! We express our love to each other many times a day and are extremely happy.

Appendix I

Senior Living Care Options

"Nothing is more difficult, and therefore more precious, than to be able to decide."
—Napoleon I (Napoleon Bonaparte), in *Napoleon's War Maxims: With His Social and Political Thoughts* (1899)

This appendix provides information about senior care facilities to help you decide what to look for when choosing a facility for yourself or others. Listed below are the major headings of this appendix.

1. Types of Senior Care Facilities
2. LivGenerations: Offerings, Fees, and Observations
3. Demystifying Assisted Living Levels and Costs
4. Examples of Other Facilities
5. Finding a Facility Meeting Your Needs

(The cost information in this appendix is specific to the facilities described. More general average cost information from many facilities is provided in Appendix II: Long-Term Care Insurance.)

Types of Senior Care Facilities

There are several types of senior living facilities. Some facilities provide only housing and housekeeping. Others provide housing, housekeeping, personal care, and medical services. Some facilities have memory care for Alzheimer's and other forms of dementia.

In an article titled "Residential Facilities, Assisted Living, and Nursing Homes,"[1] the National Institute on Aging (NIA) of the National Institutes of Health categorizes the types of facility-based long-term care services as follows: Board and Care Homes; Assisted Living Facilities; Nursing Homes; and Continuing Care Retirement Communities.

Board and Care Homes

These are small facilities where residents receive personal care and meals but not nursing or medical care. They are staffed 24 hours a day.

Assisted Living Facilities

These facilities are more comprehensive and better suited for people who need daily care. They offer different levels of care. As the required level of care increases, so does the price. These facilities do not provide nursing care. Residents have apartments or rooms and share common areas. Services generally include two or three meals a day, housekeeping, security, social activities and on-site staff. At different levels of care, making beds, taking medications, dressing, showering, and laundry can be provided.

Nursing Homes

Nursing homes provide medical care as well as the personal care services that are available in assisted living facilities. Also, they offer physical therapy, occupational therapy, wound care, intravenous (IV) therapies, and speech therapy. Most residents with chronic physical or mental conditions requiring constant care are permanent residents. Nursing homes can also be used by people who need this type of care for a short time after a hospital stay. For nursing homes in your area, search for Nursing Home Compare.[*]

Continuing Care Retirement Communities (CCRCs)

CCRCs offer different levels of service in one location. They might have stand-alone houses, but more likely apartments for independent living. You might be able to get home care in your house or apartment when needed. Typically, it would be necessary to move to a different building on the campus to receive assisted living services or nursing care. CCRDs provide medical care as well as the personal care services that are available within assisted living facilities.

LivGenerations: Offerings, Fees, and Observations

Liv is a luxury rental retirement community. It is best defined as an Assisted Living Facility. It does not provide medical care but it does have a nurse. It offers independent living, assisted living, signature care (a more comprehensive assisted living service), and memory care. Independent living and assisted living are located in one building; signature care and memory care are in another building.

One of the reasons we decided to move into a facility like LivGenerations is

---

[*] https://www.medicare.gov/nursinghomecompare/help/search-nursing-home.html.

that we can start in independent living. When we need assisted living services, we can get them without moving out of our apartment. Some senior care facilities have assisted living in a separate building. It is always challenging to move from one place to another, so this arrangement was more attractive to us.

There is a $4,000 community entrance fee but no long-term commitment. (The fee was $2,700 when we moved in.) The monthly rent includes dining, concierge service, utilities, washers and dryers in the apartments, weekly housekeeping, cable TV, high-speed internet, chauffeured transportation, wellness programs, a fitness center, and a theater.

The monthly rent includes food, but if you invite guests or eat three meals a day, you will run over the allotment paid one month in advance. There is a discounted rate for the second person in the apartment. If Jodie had to go to memory care, I would have to pay for a memory care apartment, memory care services, and separately for our current apartment because I can't live in the smaller apartments available for memory care patients.

Liv has seven one-bedroom assisted living floor plans ranging from 577 square feet to 988 square feet. Starting monthly prices range from $4,060 to $5,930 for one-person occupancy. There are two two-bedroom plans ranging from 1026 square feet to 1150 square feet. Starting monthly prices range from $6,150 to $6,705. The fee for a second occupant is $775 per month.

There are four memory care floor plans ranging from 402 square feet to 597 square feet with starting monthly prices ranging from $6,410 to $8,400. The larger size has a cost of $4,680 with shared occupancy.

We are in the larger assisted living two-bedroom apartment. Our monthly cost, paid in advance, is $ 7,538, including taxes and a covered parking space, approximately $90,500 per year. This pricing was valid in early 2020 and included a second-person fee.

We found it challenging to find an apartment with sufficient room to accommodate the needs of my special equipment to be able to shower. Having found one and knowing we could change our level of care without moving was very attractive to us. If you intend to start with independent living but think you may have to go to assisted living at some point, you should consider a facility that combines them in one building.

However, there are limitations on what services you can get with assisted living. One of my challenges is that I must be with my wife, Jodie, at all times. Having someone be with her while I went to a doctor's appointment or for any other reason is treated as "directed care" and could only be provided if I placed her in memory care.

The only other solution would be to schedule regular visits by an organization like Visiting Angels or Home Instead. Aside from the scheduling problems and the long-term commitment that would entail, I would have the same problem with Jodie's unwillingness to accept caregivers that we had in California. (As explained in the Epilogue, we were successful later in getting outside caregivers that Jodie has accepted.)

Assisted living consists of a menu of services. You choose which services you want, e.g., making your bed every day or taking out the trash every day. Our cleaning lady assessed our situation and agreed to change the sheets occasionally, which might be an assisted living service but we are not paying for it. However, I was promised they would do this before I signed a contract, so it is appropriate.

It is possible, even likely, depending on how long Jodie lives and how quickly her condition degrades, that she will need memory care. I toured the memory care building which also provides signature care. People in signature care can leave at will. The advantage of signature services is that it is less expensive than assisted living when you require more support.

That tour confirmed that we won't ever move to signature care. All the rooms in that building are too small for me and my equipment. It would not be possible for me to shower. Someone has to be with Jodie all the time. If I'm not with her, she would have to go to memory care.

Those in memory care can't leave the building unless accompanied. I try not to think about having to move Jodie into memory care because we could not live together. Separating us would crush us both. Jodie would not understand why I made that decision. She would be extremely depressed and abandoned. Worst of all, she would be convinced that I didn't love her anymore. I don't think I would be able to stand seeing her eyes, which have for so long, so perfectly, and wordlessly expressed her deep love, change to eyes showing abandonment, confusion and distress. I don't ever want to see her suffer in that way.

The only thing I could do would be to pick her up in the morning and spend the day with her before returning her to memory care at night. I would expect that she would refuse to go back into the memory care building and don't know how that would be handled.

A friend told me that, by the time she needs memory care, she might not even know who I am, so it might not be as traumatic for her. What a depressing thought! I see his point, but the implications for both of us are terribly depressing. As we have through this entire journey, we will face whatever we have to deal with and do the best we can. I acknowledge that there may be some health benefits for me to be relieved of constant care, however.

Demystifying Assisted Living Levels and Costs

Assisted living facilities offer different levels of service. It is not hard to find out what each level costs. It is unclear how to determine what level of service you need and what is included in each level. You are told that they will evaluate what you need and then assign a level to you. The problem is that you don't have any understanding of how the level is determined. Why are you in Level 3 instead of the cheaper Level 2?

As a customer, you wonder whether you need to pay for the level they chose. You are a captive customer once you join a facility, so it isn't possible to get a competitive quote. I made many attempts in various ways to learn enough about this for my own purposes and for this book. I'm not sure why most people are reluctant to give you this information. I assume that the reluctance has to do with not revealing what they consider to be competitive information.

I needed to eliminate the mystery in this process to understand what is included in the various levels of care, their cost, and how that is determined. In this chapter, I share what I have learned from a long, frustrating attempt to get this information.

I finally got some understanding of this process after I talked with the Executive Director of Liv and the Director of Sales at Sunrise of Chandler. There are at least three different methods facilities use to determine assisted living and memory levels of care services. One method is to have packages of services for each level. The complaint about that approach is that you pay for some services you don't need. Also, if you need certain kinds of care in level two and others in level three, you will pay for level three service.

The second method is to count the number of Activities of Daily Living (ADL) that the resident needs, e.g., mobility or transferring. The number of ADLs determines the level of care. That is the system Sunrise uses for all of its facilities.

Another method is a points system, which Liv uses. Each service that you need is worth a certain number of points. They add up the points for the required services. The total points determine what level you need and, therefore, what you pay. As you will see, this is a much more complex system.

I understand that Liv makes every effort to adjust down to the lower level if the total points put you just above a given level. There are six levels. Each is associated with a point range as shown below:

1. Level 1: $850   Points 1–12
2. Level 2: $1,600   Points 13–43
3. Level 3: $2,400   Points 44–62
4. Level 4: $3,200   Points 63–82
5. Level 5: $4,000   Points 83–103
6. Level 6: $4,800   Points 104+

There is also a monthly administration fee of $150.

There are seven major categories in the evaluation. I show only five below because two of them are not assigned any points. Within each category, several items are evaluated. Some of those items have no points assigned. I have listed only those items where points are assigned. For example, I list 14 items in the category, Functional Capabilities, but there are 19. No points were assigned in five of them.

Each item has multiple levels of care. For example, there are five levels of care under Eating (within the category Functional Capabilities). Two of them carry no points, and the last three have two, three and 11 possible points, respectively. I show only the minimum (two) and the maximum (11).

As my goal is to provide only the process used to select a care level, I have provided the possible points only for Functional Capabilities. However, I have shown all 58 functions that are evaluated to demonstrate the breadth of the evaluation. That information is listed below.

A. Functional Capabilities
  1. Grooming points range from three points for reminders to do it two times a day to nine points for complete assistance.
  2. Bathing points range from one point for reminders to do it two times a day to nine points for complete assistance by two caregivers for showers.
  3. Dressing points range from six points for reminders to do it up to two times a day to 17 points for complete assistance up to two times a day.
  4. Nighttime safety checks points range from two points for safety checks twice a day to six points for every two hours.
  5. Eating points range from two points for reminders to come to meals to 11 points for hand feeding.
  6. Vision costs two points for the staff to read the activity schedule and assist in planning daily schedules.
  7. Speech/communication points range from one point for requiring some repetition to six points for requiring staff assistance for communication.
  8. Mobility points range from three points for minimal physical assistance to 20 points for inability to bear weight and needs a physician confinement form.
  9. Fall risk points range from one point for limited assistance to three points for complete assistance to ambulate.
  10. Transfer ability points range from five points for one caregiver's assistance to transfer from one device to another to 23 points for assistance from two caregivers and a mechanical lift to transfer.
  11. Escorting costs eight points if you must be escorted throughout the building.
  12. Toileting points range from two points for reminders to do it two times per shift to eight points for assistance two times per shift.
  13. Hydration costs two points if you require reminders.
  14. Snacks cost one point if you require reminders.

B. Psycho/Social Capabilities
  15. to 26. Socialization/Spiritual, Transportation, Shopping, Housekeeping. Laundry, Pet Care, Smoking, Alcohol Consumption, Safety/Evacuation, Financial Affairs, Hospitality and Family Communication.

C. Cognitive Capabilities
  27. to 34. Cognition, Cognitive Stimulation, Behavior, Mood, Time/Place Orientation, Wandering, Anxiety and Personal Safety.

D. Special Medical Needs
  35. to 51. Oxygen, Breathing Treatments, Diabetes, Skin Care, Healing Wounds, Indwelling Urinary Catheter, Injections, Colostomy/ileostomy, Hospice, Weight Loss/Gain, Lab Work, Vital Signs, Coordination of Care,

Pain, Bed Mobility Device, Physical Therapy and Occupational Therapy (PT/OT) and Home Health Nurse.

E. Medication Management

52. to 58. Oral Medication, Special Medications Treatments, Medication Setup, Medication Storage, MAR/Meds Review, Pharmacy and Crush Medications.

The assessment involves the resident deciding what they want and the facility determining what the individual needs. For example, the individual might decide he or she doesn't want to be escorted, but if that involves an unacceptable safety risk, escorting would be included.

While the attempt is to be very specific on each factor, there is a range of points possible for each factor, so there is still a degree of judgment that can affect the selected level. I believe that is why Liv makes an effort to select a lower level when the result of the assessment is at the lower end of a level.

Examples of Other Facilities

Sunrise of Chandler*

Chandler, Arizona, borders Phoenix and is close to LivGenerations. Sunrise of Chandler is a part of Sunrise Senior Living which operates more than 325 communities throughout the U.S., Canada and the United Kingdom, making it the 5th largest senior living provider in the U.S. Sunrise Senior Living collectively offers assisted living, personal care, independent living, Alzheimer's & memory care, skilled nursing & rehabilitative care, and short-term stays.

Pamela, the Director of Sales, was very helpful. Not only did she provide all the information I wanted about Sunrise, she asked questions about our situation and needs. Realizing that I needed a caregiver that could come for a few hours as needed, she sent me a brochure of a company that would meet that need. I was convinced that Sunrise could help Jodie with showers after talking with Pamela, something I haven't accomplished. Unfortunately, given the size of my wheelchair and other special equipment, the suite sizes are too small for me.

Sunrise of Chandler provides assisted living and memory care. As a part of your rental, they offer three meals a day, daily trash removal, weekly housekeeping, weekly laundry service, monthly visits by a licensed nurse, and scheduled transportation. This facility is highly rated.

The suites do not have washers and dryers. They offer weekly laundry service for personal laundry, linens and towels. If that is insufficient, there are laundry rooms that the residents can use.

Sunrise doesn't have any two-bedroom, two-bath suites. Relative to Liv, the suites are small. The largest suite is 525 square feet. It is a one-bedroom/Den. The largest that Liv offers is 1150 square feet, the smallest is 577 square feet.

Sunrise has a move-in fee of $2,500. Other fees are listed below.

---

* https://www.sunriseseniorliving.com/communities/sunrise-of-chandler/about.aspx.

Assisted Living Fees

Suite Rates Starting at:	Daily	Monthly	Yearly
Companion Living Suite	$95	$2,889	$34,675
Studio Suite	$125	$3,802	$45,625
One Bedroom	$145	$4,410	$52,925
Two Bedroom/One Bath	$148	$4,502	$54,020
Care Level Rates Starting at:	Daily	Monthly	Yearly
Assisted Living Select (1-2 ADLs)	$23	$700	$8,395
Assisted Living Plus (3-4 ADLs)	$45	$1,369	$16,425
Assisted Living Plus Plus (5-8 ADLs)	$79	$2,403	$28,835
Enhanced Care (9-12 ADLs)	$79	$2,403	$28,835
Additional Services Starting at:	Daily	Monthly	Yearly
Medication Level 1 1-6 Meds	$17	$517	$6,205
Medication Level 2 7-9 Meds	$22	$669	$8,030
Medication Level 3 10+ Meds, Inj, Inh*	$28	$852	$10,220

* 10+ Medications or any injections or inhalers.

Sunrise doesn't consider that they offer independent living, but effectively they do. If you don't need any personal care, your only charge is for your suite. Recognizing that these are "starting at" prices, the annual cost for a two-bedroom, one-bath suite would be as low as $54,020. Prices vary depending on location, size of suite and view. As mentioned earlier, the level of personal care that applies is based on the number of Activities of Daily Living (ADL). The seven types of ADLs are mobility, transferring, grooming, showering, toileting, dressing and dining.

If you need an ADL, e.g., transferring, it doesn't matter how many times you use it. For example, if you need assistance with mobility four times daily and six transfers, you would be in Assisted Living Select because that would be two ADLs. You are charged an additional ADL if two care managers are needed for the transfers. The same is true with showers. If two care managers are needed for a weekly shower, you are charged with two ADLs instead of one. Two to three showers per week are two ADLs and four or more showers a week are three ADLs.

Memory Care Fees

Suite Rates Starting at:	Daily	Monthly	Yearly
Companion Living Suite	$90	$2,738	$32,850
Studio Suite	$115	$3,498	$41,975
One Bedroom	$138	$4,198	$50,370
Two Bedroom/One Bath	$145	$4,410	$52,925
Care Level Rates Starting at:	Daily	Monthly	Yearly
Assisted Living Select (0-4 ADLs)*	$57	$1,734	$20,805
Assisted Living Plus (5-8 ADLs)	$89	$2,707	$32,485
Assisted Living Plus Plus (9-12 ADLs)	$120	$3,650	$43,800
Enhanced Care (13+ ADLs)	$140	$4,258	$51,100

Additional Fees:	(Medication)	Daily	Monthly	Yearly
Medication Level 1	1-6 Meds	$21	$517	$6,205
Medication Level 2	7-9 Meds	$26	$669	$8,030
Medication Level 3	10+ Meds, Inj, Inh**	$32	$852	$10,220

* Note that when living in memory care, the minimum of care fee is $20,805 even if you do not need any assistance, a very unlikely possibility.
** Any injections or inhalations automatically put you in Medication Level 3.

Bay Woods of Annapolis*

My fraternity brother, Fred Hellrich, told me about two CCRCs located in the Annapolis, Maryland, area near his home, Bay Woods of Annapolis and The Village at Providence Point. I am providing information on both of them to show that many different facilities offer senior living.

Fred's wife received comprehensive care at Bay Woods of Annapolis, a Continuing Care Retirement Community, for seven weeks of rehabbing due to hip replacement surgery complications. As mentioned earlier, some facilities offer short-term care for people after a hospital stay. Bay Woods is different from most facilities in that it is a resident-owned and resident-run co-operative community. Below are some excerpts from Fred's observations from this experience.

> They operate all levels of service/care.... They reserve a certain number of rooms for comprehensive care for their residents, but accept short term rehab patients ... when room is available. We had to pay an entrance fee to become members of the Co-op, even though Mary was a short term patient. The fee was $11,000 but it is refundable when leaving the facility. Mary's Comprehensive Care cost was $372/day, which is in the range for most facilities around here. Mary was private pay, with the additional medical services (therapy, doctors, etc.) paid for by her Medicare and her secondary insurance.
>
> I can't praise enough the total operation of the facility. She had a comparatively large private room with a full private bath. All services were provided in the room (bathing, dining when she was not up to going to the dining room), large screen TV, full cable TV including Hulu, all carpeted floors, restaurant style menu for choosing all of her meals, a full slate of activities to choose from and more. The food was good and excellently prepared.

Fred's wife was in a different rehab facility for physical therapy for a week after a previous surgery. The experience there was very different. It was essentially a hospital-style environment with a semi-private room, non-carpeted floors, and only a shared half bath with the room next door. Bathing was down the hall in a non-private shower room.

After experiencing two different facilities for the same purpose, Fred said, "It was an eye-opener to me to see how the comprehensive care units differ among retirement communities. How they are run may be more important than how the independent living facility is...."

Bay Woods is a co-op; residents collectively own the land and buildings through a co-operative housing corporation. Their equity position creates income tax deductions and possible capital gains or losses. Residents are responsible for

---

* https://www.baywoodsofannapolis.com/documents/2020%20Brochure%20(003).pdf.

the overall operation of Bay Woods, including the annual budget, approval of the monthly fees, and capital improvements decisions.

The 2020 entrance fee is $15,460. Unit size ranges from 980 to 2,480 square feet. Monthly fees range from $3,718 to $5,436 for the first person and average $1,033 for the second.

In addition to the usual service expected in a senior care facility like meals and housekeeping, other services include: licensed nurses; acute medical condition care; physical therapy; occupational therapy; speech therapy; physicians on-call; physician-ordered diagnostic procedures including x-rays, labs, etc.; stroke recovery; licensed certified social worker; terminal illness care; diabetic care; pharmacy services; blood pressure checks; dermatological services; podiatrist visits; and dentist visits.

The Village at Providence Point*

The Village at Providence Point is a Continuing Care Retirement Community (CCRC) in Annapolis, Maryland. Cottages and apartment homes are on a wooded campus, located 10 minutes from Annapolis, a high-cost area. It is a not-for-profit, faith-based National Lutheran Community that is projected to open in 2023. They accept refundable $1,000 deposits, which reserves a position for selecting a cottage or an apartment.

You commit to rent a living unit by paying either an entrance fee that is 50 percent refundable on leaving or 90 percent refundable on leaving. In the information below, the lower fee is 50 percent refundable, the higher fee is 90 percent refundable. A commitment to rent a unit guarantees the 2023 pricing. Living facility options are listed below.

1. One-bedroom apartments with one and a half baths. Apartment size ranges from 920 to 1,050 square feet. The associated entrance fee ranges from $319,000 (50 percent refundable) to $740,400 (90 percent refundable). Monthly rent ranges from $3,100 to $3,571.
2. Two-bedroom apartments with two baths. Apartment size ranges from 1,200 to 1,745 square feet. The associated entrance fee ranges from $429,812 to $1,228,000. Monthly rent ranges from $4,100 to $5,925.
3. Penthouse. 1,950 square feet. The associated entrance fee ranges from $720,276 to $1,374,968. Monthly rent is $6,632.
4. Two-bedroom cottages. Cottage size ranges from 2,040 to 2,540 square feet. The associated entrance fee ranges from $536,100 to $1,334,059. Monthly rent ranges from $3,680 to $4,600.

The second-person entrance fee is $35,000, and the monthly fee is $1,000.

The next step in reserving a spot in Providence Point occurs when it gets State approval to operate, at which time a 10 percent refundable down payment is made.

---

* www.thevillageatprovidencepoint.org/our-community.

Brookdale Facilities

Brookdale was the first senior care company that I encountered. While we were living in Danville, California, we frequently drove by and walked past Brookdale Diablo Lodge, an assisted living facility. It was near the end of our short street and on our walking path. We had a friend who lived there. When my wife, Jodie, declined rapidly in July 2019, we visited this facility because I hoped she could stay there at night and come home during the day. Sometimes she could remain in Brookdale while I spent some time with my friends. Diablo Lodge decided she needed to go to Brookdale Danville, a memory care facility. It was a short drive from our home in the same town. I visited Brookdale Danville with John from my golf group. I wasn't ready to put Jodie in memory care. Soon after that, we decided to move to Arizona.

Brookdale is the largest of the senior care facilities in the United States. Collectively their facilities offer independent living, assisted living, memory care, continuing care retirement communities and skilled nursing. Specific facilities usually provide only one or two of these services. What they offer depends on what plan they developed for that site and the license they obtained from the state.

Based on my research on many of the Brookdale facilities in the Chandler area, their living spaces are smaller than those available at Liv. Many of them are highly rated and could be of interest to others. However, considering that I have a sizeable motorized wheelchair and need special equipment for showering and toiletry, I would not be able to live in them. More details on living space sizes are provided below.

The method for determining the appropriate level of assisted living required is similar to the system Sunrise uses, i.e., points are assigned based on the number of the various types of care used, not how often they are used, except in a few instances.

Brookdale Chandler Ray Road offers secured assisted living. I had not heard of secured assisted living before. You cannot leave the facility without someone from the organization opening the door for you. They have six floor plans ranging from 288 square feet to 443 square feet. They have no two-bedroom floor plans.

Brookdale Chandler Regional offers both assisted living and independent living. They have eleven floor plans ranging from 291 square feet to 780 square feet. They have one plan with two bedrooms that is 737 square feet.

Brookdale Central Chandler has both assisted living and memory care. All apartments are shared except for the smallest. They have three floor plans ranging from 240 square feet to 360 square feet. The average size is 340 square feet. Most likely, Jodie and I could not stay in the same apartment in this facility. We would each have to share our room with some unrelated party.

An evaluation of the appropriate level of assisted care is made by the nurse based on the worst day of the evaluation period. Evaluation occurs after 14, 30, and 60 days, and quarterly thereafter. The price you pay could go up or down after an evaluation.

Brookdale Springs Mesa offers independent living & assisted living. There are only two floor plans. The one-bedroom floor plan has 625 square feet and the two-bedroom floor plan 825 square feet.

Brookdale Santa Catalina, Tucson. In searching for a facility that has more than two types of care, I found this facility in Tucson, over 100 miles away. It offers independent living, assisted living, memory care, continuing care retirement community and skilled nursing.

Finding a Facility Meeting Your Needs

When you start searching for a facility in your area, there are several ways to proceed. I found that searching for senior living facilities on Google Maps was effective. Google will plot facility locations near where you wish to live on a map. By placing your mouse on a facility, you will get the name of the facility, a picture of it, the type of care they offer, and a star rating.

Another approach is to use "A Place for Mom."[*] They will require you to give your name, email, phone number, type of care needed, and zip code before they will help.

Another approach is to go to the websites of some of the largest caregiving firms. By filling out a form on the companies' websites and choosing a state, city or zip code, the type of care facility of interest, and the maximum distance from your desired location, options and locations for that company's facilities will be displayed. The drawback is that only that firm's facilities will be shown.

Several large senior living firms will possibly have a facility near you. Generations is listed in the top 125 largest senior caregiving firms. Within a few miles of Generations, Brookdale and Sunrise both have facilities. As mentioned earlier, Brookdale is the largest. Sunrise is the second largest in some categories. To assist you in that process, listed below is information on some of the largest firms. The footnotes provide website addresses.

An article by Elizabeth Ecker in *Senior Housing News* titled "Largest Senior Living Provider List Grows in 2018"[2] provides a ranking of the largest senior care facilities in the U.S. This information was generated by Argentum,[3] the leading national trade association serving companies that own, operate, and support professionally managed senior living communities in the United States.

The ranking for the top five number of units by category is shown below. To demonstrate the dominance of Brookdale, I have listed the number of units for the top two in each category.

Total Units

1. Brookdale Senior Living[†]   80,526 units
2. Holiday Retirement[‡]   31,731 units

---

[*] www.aplaceformom.com.
[†] https://www.brookdale.com/en.html.
[‡] https://www.holidaytouch.com/.

3. Life Care Services[*]
4. Five Star Senior Living[†]
5. Sunrise Senior Living

Assisted Living

1. Brookdale Senior Living   49,740 units
2. Sunrise Senior Living   14,615 units
3. Five Star Senior Living
4. Altria Senior Living[‡]
5. Senior Lifestyle Corp[§]

Independent Living

1. Holiday Retirement   30,839 units
2. Brookdale Senior Living   27,888 units
3. Life Care Services
4. Erickson Living
5. Five Star Senior Living

Memory Care

1. Brookdale Senior Living   12,888 units
2. Sunrise Senior Living   5,683 units
3. Five Star Senior Living
4. ALG Senior[¶]
5. Senior Lifestyle Corp

Closing

Fred Hellrich did some research on the performance of some of the facilities his wife used regarding COVID-19 and reported:

> The recent facility Mary was at had two workers and two residents testing positive for COVID-19 and no deaths. The facility Mary stayed at previously had many more cases and several deaths. I attribute that to the fact that Mary's recent facility had all private rooms, private baths and in-room meal service. The other facility did not, including common showering facilities. In fact, one of the articles in the paper cited the fact that nursing homes with non-private facilities was a significant issue in the terrible contraction rates in nursing homes. Also, I am sure, how aggressive the facility enforced anti-contagion procedures was a factor. But certainly, in choosing a nursing facility, one should factor in how well it performed for this pandemic.

Liv had no infections of the virus among residents or staff at the time I wrote the Appendix. We hope never to have another pandemic, but our seasonal viruses

---

[*] https://www.lifecareservices-seniorliving.com/.
[†] https://www.fivestarseniorliving.com/.
[‡] https://www.atriaseniorliving.com/.
[§] https://www.seniorlifestyle.com/.
[¶] https://www.algsenior.com/.

cause many deaths. Learning how well the facilities you are considering performed should be factored into your decision process.

The information in this appendix will help you find some options for senior
living in the area of your choice. Reading their literature and visiting them first
by a virtual tour and then in person will help you chose the best facility for your
needs and desires.

Appendix II

Long-Term Care Insurance

"It's better to be boldly decisive and risk being wrong than to agonize at length and be right too late."
—Marilyn Moats Kennedy, "The Case Against
Performance Appraisals," in *Across the Board* (January 1999)

Developing severe disabilities requiring long-term care is one of the most significant financial risks facing the elderly. For many older people, the cost of long-term care facilities is unaffordable. For that reason, if you are over 50 years old, you should consider long-term care insurance. Once you have a debilitating condition, you will not qualify for it.

This type of insurance is valuable when you have a chronic or progressive medical condition, e.g., nerve disease, muscle disease, or dementia. Other types of insurance, including Medicare, don't cover long-term care. Medicare covers only limited home health care which does not include day-to-day help. Most long-term care policies will reimburse you for care in your home and senior living facilities, including assisted living or memory care.

For traditional long-term care policies, you will pay an annual premium covering financial assistance for day-to-day activities such as showering, bathing, getting in and out of bed, etc. Most policies won't pay benefits unless you cannot perform at least two daily living activities without help, or you have dementia or another cognition disability. They also generally require you to pay for the first 30 to 90 days. These policies typically have both a daily limit and a lifetime maximum. Some policies pay less if your facility doesn't have a nurse 24 hours a day.

If you don't have insurance to cover long-term care, you'll have to pay for it yourself. Those with low incomes can get help through Medicaid, the federal and state health insurance program, but only after you've exhausted most of your savings. Long-term care insurance is necessary if you don't have sufficient assets to pay for living in a senior living facility or wish to preserve your assets.

When I started looking at senior living facilities, I got an appreciation for how expensive they are. We are in independent living at LivGenerations. The annual cost is over $90,000 per year. Appendix I: Senior Living Care Options provides more information on senior living alternatives' types and costs.

We never bought long-term care insurance because of my financial philosophy. While we were young and had limited assets, I decided to self-insure for everything except home insurance, auto insurance, and life insurance. This included extended warranties. I believed that, as long as I could cover immediate emergencies, we would be better off in the long run. It has served us well. Partly as a result, we can incur the cost of senior living for a long time.

I recommend that you read "A Shopper's Guide to Long-Term Care Insurance" by the National Association of Insurance Commissioners[1] if you decide to consider purchasing long-term care insurance. The guide covers every subject that might be of interest regarding long-term care insurance. Consider their rule of thumb "[I]t should cost less than 7% of your income" when deciding whether you can afford it.

New York Life Insurance Company has an article titled "Long-Term Care: Plan for the Future" on an AARP website[2] that provides some useful information about the possible need for insurance and the cost of it. Here are some of the key points that they make:

1. [E]ven the most well-thought-out plans may not be enough to prepare you for the unexpected costs associated with long-term care.
2. 70% of people turning 65 can expect to use some form of long-term care during their lives.
3. Nursing Home Care: The average cost of a year's care in a private Medicare-certified long-term nursing home room is $104,000.
4. Home Care: The average in-home care costs $49,920 a year for 40 hours of help per week.
5. Assisted Living Care: A year in a 1-bedroom assisted living care facility averages $57,000 per year.

Another good source of information about long-term care insurance is an article by Barbara Marquand in NerdWallet dated May 28, 2019, "Long-Term Care Insurance Explained." NerdWallet[3] provides these examples of the cost of long-term care insurance:

> A single 55-year-old man ... can expect to pay an average of $2,050 a year ... with an initial pool of benefits of $164,000.... For the same policy, a single 55-year-old woman can expect to pay an average of $2,700 a year. The average combined premiums for a 55-year-old couple ... are $3,050 a year.

The U.S. Department of Health and Human Services, through the Office of the Assistant Secretary for Planning and Evaluation, in conjunction with the Urban Institute, prepared the report "Long-Term Services and Supports for Older Americans: Risks and Financing Research Brief."[4] They concluded that "most Americans underestimate the risk of developing a disability and needing long-term services.... Most will need assistance for less than two years. About one in seven adults, however, will have a disability for more than five years. On average, an American turning 65 today will incur $138,000 in future ... costs."

I mentioned that the terms of the policies discussed so far refer to "traditional" long-term care policies. But there are newer hybrid policies that combine life insurance with long-term care.* This is because there is considerable risk for both the insurer and the insured with traditional policies.

Ellen Stark makes this point in the bulletin she prepared for AARP, "5 Things You SHOULD Know About Long-Term Care Insurance."[5] One of her main points is that traditional policies have an unfortunate history.

> Typical terms today [2018] include a daily benefit of $160 for nursing home coverage, a waiting period of about three months before insurance kicks in and a maximum of three years' worth of coverage.... [They] have had a troubled history of premium spikes and insurer losses, thanks in part to faulty forecasts by insurers of the amount of care they'd be on the hook for. Sales have fallen sharply. While more than 100 insurers sold policies in the 1990s, now fewer than 15 do.

This is due to the uncertain cost of future claims and low-interest rates. Insurers invest the premiums; low-interest rates reduce their returns. State regulators allow the insurance companies to increase their rates because they fear that the insurance companies might not have sufficient funds to continue paying claims and declare bankruptcy or stop selling insurance if they don't. The reduction in firms offering this type of insurance demonstrates that this risk is real.

Stark makes the point that you can draw from the hybrid whole life insurance policy for long-term care. "Unlike the older variety of ... insurance, these 'hybrid' policies will return money to your heirs even if you don't end up needing long-term care. With these policies, you don't risk a rate hike associated with traditional policies' because you lock in your premium upfront. Also, if you're older or have health problems, you may be more likely to qualify."[6]

These policies cost two or three times that of traditional policies. You have to weigh the higher cost versus eliminating the risk of future rate hikes and the lower risk of your insurer declaring bankruptcy, plus the other benefits you will gain by purchasing a hybrid policy.

Another source of cost information is Genworth's Cost of Care Survey 2019.[7] Genworth's website includes a Care Survey tool to allow you to estimate the annual median cost for various types of care. The price of the rooms is based on a single room. Here is some information from Genworth: "Every day until 2030, 10,000 Baby Boomers will turn 65 and 7 out of 10 people will require long term care in their lifetime. The cost of that care varies based on the care setting, geographic location of care and level of care required, among other things."

The decision process regarding whether to purchase a policy for long-term care insurance is complex and multifaceted. The same is true for when to do so and the choice between traditional and hybrid policies. The information appearing in this appendix should guide you through making a decision that is compatible with your situation.

---

* Search for Brighthouse SmartCare® hybrid insurance for an example.

Appendix III

Documents Your Heirs Will Need

"Success depends upon previous preparation, and without such preparation there is sure to be failure."

—*Confucius*

Thinking about and planning for your demise is not an uplifting task. For many people, it is not a subject they are willing to address. Just talking about it disturbs our daughter, Kris. However, your responsibility is to provide the information that your family will need when you are gone. It is essential if you are a caregiver for someone who would need immediate attention. A severe medical condition or near accident will often cause individuals to realize the importance of this planning; don't wait for that!

Arie J. Korving, in his book *Before I Go: Preparing Your Affairs for Your Heirs*,[1] describes the intense period of grief, anger, confusion, and fear felt by the wife of someone he knew when her husband died. Her husband had taken care of everything while he lived, and she was not prepared to manage her affairs after he died. You want to avoid this outcome for your heirs.

Don't procrastinate!! It's too important. Regardless of how healthy you feel and how busy you are, none of us are guaranteed tomorrow. Start now taking these end-of-life steps, even though it sounds daunting. Starting with the most crucial information and then taking on one subject at a time will give you a sense of accomplishment. This appendix suggests the subjects and content of the documents needed to provide vital information for your heirs. It contains recommendations regarding the legal and general information documents you should prepare for your family and heirs. For an extensive treatment of end-of-life planning, I recommend *A Beginner's Guide to the End: Practical Advice for Living Life and Facing Death* by B.J. Miller and Shoshana Berger.[2] Chapter One is titled "Don't Leave a Mess."[3] The title makes it clear that a responsible person will do what they can to minimize the effort and anguish that your survivors will face. Following the suggestions in this section will help to avoid those issues.

Legal Documents

I recommend that you have an estate attorney prepare the following documents:

1. Durable powers of attorney for health care
2. Powers of attorney for financial matters
3. A living trust with successor trustees
4. Advance health care directive
5. Authorizations to release health information protected by the Health Insurance Portability & Accountability Act (HIPAA)
6. Conventional wills

You can find do-it-yourself forms for these documents on the Internet, but an estate attorney is better prepared to create them. State laws vary and circumstances change. A periodic review is also advisable.

General Information Documents

Preparing legal documents is very important, but they are not everything that the family will need. You should also prepare general information documents for those left behind. A listing of the recommended materials follows:

1. Immediate Action
2. Family, Friends, and Neighbors' Contact Information
3. Passwords
4. Financial Records
5. Death Notices
6. Retirement Accounts, Pensions, and Social Security
7. Medical Information
8. Brokerage and Mutual Fund Accounts
9. Banks
10. Credit Cards
11. Insurance Policies
12. Taxes
13. Selling Assets
14. Private Stock
15. Lawyers
16. Art

These subjects can be covered in separate documents or combined in ways that make sense for your situation. For each topic I discuss, provide the following contact information: Agent name, address, e-mail, and phone numbers; account numbers; insurance IDs; group numbers; and any additional relevant information needed for others to take the necessary action.

To ensure that required payments are made on time to avoid loss of services, insurance, penalties, and interest charges, as many transactions as possible should happen automatically. Immediate action on the part of your heirs and the effort required to maintain the everyday activities of life will thus be minimized.

Immediate Action

While we lived in California, a long way from our family, immediate action would be needed because Jodie could not be left alone for even 30 minutes. I listed family contact information for those friends and neighbors who would care for her until a family member could arrive. My family would be notified of my death by a neighbor or by first responders. A 911 call made from my phone would display family names and phone numbers because of Smart911 discussed in Chapter 12, How to Prepare for Emergencies. As we have since moved near family, this concern no longer exists for us, but if your situation is similar to what ours was while we lived in California, you should consider the same action.

If you have rental storage, provide all the information they might need to access it.

Family, Friends, and Neighbors' Contact Information

To enable rapid communications, I provided documents to friends and neighbors, listing contacts for my extended family. Similarly, my family has contact information for friends and neighbors.

Passwords

For most people, your computer provides access to your most important documents and accounts. Examples include banks, mutual funds, brokerage accounts, income tax software (e.g., TurboTax), state and federal tax payment websites, utility accounts, financial software (e.g., Quicken), insurance accounts, shopping websites, health care, airlines, and more. Because hackers are always seeking this information, you should utilize complex passwords to access these accounts. But complex passwords become a big problem if you haven't provided a way for your heirs to locate them in your absence. Like the example mentioned above from Arie Korving's book, this issue was impressed on me by a real-life example. A relative of a friend unexpectedly died at a young age. He had used complex passwords, and no one had access to them, thus creating significant family complications.

For that reason, a document, or series of documents, should be prepared wherein IDs and passwords for important accounts can be found. There are many ways to accomplish this. The choice I made utilizes multiple security measures. Getting access to sign-in information requires accessing two password-protected documents, neither of which directly provides that information. There is a key the family knows well that is needed to decode the information in those documents.

These documents also contain routing numbers and account numbers for bank accounts. This information can be used to allow funds transfer between banks and between banks and investment accounts. It can also be used to pay income taxes.

While I remember many IDs and passwords, it is more efficient when you are working on the computer to use something like Norton Identify Safe. The documents discussed above could be used by the family to find the password for Norton Identify Safe, which would be helpful if they had access to my computer.

Financial Records

I recommend that you provide a document containing critical financial information. Most won't want to go as far as I did. I have a massive spreadsheet containing many years of financial information, including total assets at the end of each year, all purchases, sales, dividend reinvestments, and much more information than I will discuss here.

Quicken[*] and Morningstar[†] are other ways to keep financial information. They have the advantage of easily being updated to be current, unlike the spreadsheet where pricing must be entered. Morningstar is online and is suitable for stocks and mutual funds. It shows the current value and change in the value of individual holdings and your total portfolio. It also can show how your assets are distributed among types of assets. Some mutual fund companies will cover the cost of Morningstar Premium.

Quicken resides on your computer and can show the current value of your total portfolio. It also provides balances and transactions for your banks, credit cards, mutual funds, and stocks. You can also initiate payments from it. Because of the detailed record of transactions, it is a great way to search for information needed for income tax preparation. It is also valuable for determining when you bought an item and its cost. I use it frequently for that purpose.

Even Excel can be used to maintain records of purchases. An Excel file for each year, listing all tax-related purchases, payments, and check numbers, when a check was used, can facilitate tax preparation.

Death Notices

Many organizations will need a death notice, and some will require certified copies, e.g., Medicare, Medicare Supplement insurance, Social Security, life insurance policies, and pensions. Provide information on how to obtain certified death certificates and who would need them. The funeral home you're working with can get certified copies on your behalf. Generally, you can also get them from your county health department and the county recorder. Discuss requirements with your estate attorney as he/she will have up-to-date information.

---

[*] https://www.quicken.com/.
[†] https://www.morningstar.com/.

Retirement Accounts, Pensions, and Social Security

If you are required to make Minimum Required Distributions (MRDs), mutual funds holding your retirement funds can help you determine the amount and when the final MRD will have to be paid. They will create an inherited IRA, from which additional MRD payments will have to be made. I recommend setting up automatic payments for the MRD in December of each year. Explain how to ensure there is sufficient cash available at that time to pay the MRD. Otherwise, the mutual fund will do it in a way that might not be as advantageous to your heirs. Explain where pension payments are paid and remind them to notify the company to discontinue payments. Social Security will pay a small one-time death benefit. If your Social Security payment is more substantial than your spouse's, their payment will increase to the higher amount you were getting.

Medical Information

All doctors who attend to a member of the household should be identified. Create separate medical history documents for each of you. These documents should include current medications (including frequency and dosage), past and current medical conditions, blood pressure, vitamins, eyesight, vaccines, surgeries, past medications, and allergies. It is important to include family medical history and conditions (e.g., mother died from lung cancer, brother has both an ascending and a descending aorta aneurysm) when they are known.

Brokerage and Mutual Fund Accounts

Identify those accounts that are included in your trust and those that are not. (I recommend that all significant assets be placed in your trust to avoid probate court issues.) I have always maintained a balanced investment account and weighted investments toward mutual funds to limit risk. If you are an active investor, consider changing your investment philosophy. To avoid the need for immediate action when you can no longer manage them, consolidate stocks and mutual funds into a minimum number of accounts. Increase the percentage of your assets in cash. Have all distributions paid in cash. Preferably, have them auto-transferred into your highest interest-bearing account. Internet banks pay a higher interest rate. Link investment accounts to all banks and adjust the settings, so any sales or income proceeds are automatically transferred to the bank of your choice. Otherwise, the investment account will pay a very low-interest rate on cash.

Banks

Most people have a regular bank used for depositing funds, writing checks, and possibly a safe deposit box. If this account is not in the trust, deposits in them should be modest to avoid probate. List automatic payments into this bank, e.g., pension, and withdrawals, e.g., Medicare Supplemental insurance, and the dates they occur. This information helps determine what balance should be maintained. Provide the location of your checkbooks.

If you have a safe deposit box, advise the family where to locate the key. You should have one or more of your heirs authorized to access the box. Do this when the family is in town.* Have them empty the box before the bank is notified of your death to avoid delayed access. The bank can/will freeze access to your box when they are notified of your death.

You might use Internet banks due to the higher interest rate they pay. If you have more than one, I recommend that you connect them so you can transfer funds via the Automated Clearing House (ACH) process.† You should also connect them to your regular bank and your financial accounts. Money can then easily be transferred wherever it is needed. Note that only six withdraws are permitted per month from Internet banks. List the closing date for each account and any automatic withdrawals or deposits associated with that bank. This will help ensure that your heirs don't exceed the six withdrawals limit in the monthly accounting period used by your bank(s). Each bank uses its own accounting period. If you are required to pay Federal and state income taxes electronically, provide information on scheduling them through the U.S. Treasury and state websites. If you keep a much larger balance in Internet banks, you will likely use an Internet bank to pay those taxes. Suggest which to use. Inform your family that the amount of FDIC coverage will change after your death. The balances in each account should be checked against the new limit.

Credit Cards

Provide a list of which credit card accounts you own and automatic payments made from them. If the credit card balance is paid automatically, list the account that makes the payment. Pay as many bills as possible with the credit card to reduce the number of withdrawals from banks, the number of checks needed, the required balance in the regular bank, and to build up airline mileage or cash credit. Let your family know which credit cards have airline mile credits or cash rebates associated with them. Your accounts should be canceled but caution the family that the airline miles will expire two years from that date.

Insurance Policies

Provide the names of insurance companies used for life, health, home, earthquake, auto, flood, and liability policies. Include when they are due, IDs, account numbers, and how they are paid (preferably auto paid). Advise your heirs to

---

* There is a way to remotely register family members for your safe deposit box, but everyone has to be in a branch of the bank simultaneously and a time must be established that works with all involved branches of the bank.

† An ACH transfer is an electronic, bank-to-bank means of transferring funds for person-to-person payments, bill payments and direct deposits from employers and government benefit programs.

contact all insurance companies for processing claims, e.g., life insurance, making necessary adjustments, e.g., fewer drivers for auto insurance or cancellation, e.g., health insurance. If the cost of prescription plans under Medicare are automatically deducted from your Social Security payments, so note. If you use online drug companies associated with Medicare Part D to get a 90 day supply, include that information. If you have burial and funeral insurance, supply that information.

Taxes

Your family will need (1) access to prior tax returns, (2) the data used to create your returns, (3) to know whether you engaged an accountant or used tax preparation software, and (4) to know whether you are required to pay federal and state income taxes electronically. Estimated income tax payments are due quarterly. I use TurboTax and save PDF copies on the computer. If you have a significant account with some firms like T. Rowe Price, you will get TurboTax at a discount. When I prepared my 2019 returns, the year we moved, I used the online, Premier version of TurboTax because I earned money from rental income and had capital gains. Premium tax software can import your investment information, but I prefer to insert the data myself. I paid nothing for using the software, filing a two-state tax return, and electronically filing the returns. If you used an accountant or believe your heirs would need to, identify or suggest an accountant.

Include information on where copies of the returns are located and where to find the data used to prepare the returns, e.g., 1099 INT forms. If they decide to use itemized deductions, explain where other necessary information can be found. In my case, Quicken can be used for that purpose. After the Tax Cuts and Jobs Act was enacted in 2017, the standard deduction nearly doubled. For that reason, I have found that itemization is not necessary. In the document on banks, I explained how to make electronic tax payments. You might want to repeat that information in this document if it applies.

The document should list taxes associated with any homes or land you own, when they are due, and what they cost. If there are tax advantages to paying in one payment instead of multiple payments, make that suggestion.

Selling Assets

Make suggestions concerning your home, vehicles, property, and equipment, which would no longer be needed or which would create an unneeded burden. In my case, I offered three options for our home. It could be sold, rented, or left vacant. I discussed the estate tax advantage of not selling it and what would be required to leave it unoccupied or to rent it. If they keep the house, they will need names and contact information for services like the gardener, cleaning lady, handyman, and contractor. Whatever the family decides, they need to know where to find the title insurance policy.

I recommended selling my handicap-equipped van. Firms that sell and install hand controls to create handicapped vehicles maintain an inventory of vans. They have customers with budget concerns, so they sell used vans as well as new ones. I suggested companies that would be potential buyers. I suggested that the SUV would be an excellent vehicle for the family to keep, but the rear scooter lift should be removed to increase rear window visibility. Make sure to let your family know where to find the vehicle titles.

I mentioned that an undeveloped property we own in another state should be sold. The lifts in the house could be sold back to the company that sold them to me. eBay would be another option. My scooter and wheelchair could be sold on eBay.

Private Stock

If you own private stock, provide the company names, contact information and stock certificate locations.

Lawyers

If you are using a lawyer(s), or have used them in the past, provide the firm names, the specific lawyers you engaged, the purpose, and contact information. This is very important if the lawyers have not yet completed the task assigned to them.

Art

If you have purchased original art, you might have saved information about it, including the date of purchase, the original price, and the receipt. Make sure you specify where that information is stored. If you want to establish who gets the art, include that information in your will.

The documents suggested herein will be a guide. Preparing all these documents might seem like a daunting task, but if you take them one at a time, you will continue to make progress and be encouraged to continue. Start with the most important documents first.

The references I have provided discuss issues like a letter to the family if you feel you haven't conveyed your love for them adequately or have specific wishes like funeral arrangements or church services.

As you complete the documents, you need to find a way to ensure that your heirs can have ready access to them. The next appendix offers some alternative methods.

Appendix IV

Ready Document Access Is a Must

*"Don't just be a giver. Be an extremely helpful giver who demonstrates
an awareness of what that person most needs."*
—Kare Anderson, in *Mutuality Matters* (2014)

Preparing the documents mentioned in Appendix III is the most time-consuming task when preparing your heirs for your death, but quick access to up-to-date versions of these documents is vital. This is particularly true when your family is remote from your location. Appendix IV offers optional methods for granting ready access to these documents. Many ways to accomplish this and the pros and cons of each approach are discussed in this appendix. I have used all of the options mentioned below.

The simplest way to make the documents available is to print them or copy them to a thumb drive. Then you can give your heirs the copies or drives when you see them or send them via mail. This is a relatively secure and straightforward approach. However, the information is likely to be out of date when needed. Also, your heirs might not remember where they have placed documents when they need them. They could place them in a safe deposit box or a fireproof file cabinet, but this method shares the concern about potentially being out of date when needed. Ready access to them could also be problematic.

There are programs like Send Anywhere that will allow you to send your documents securely. However, you have to keep posting updates as you modify the materials. Frequent modification is not an issue with the legal documents, but it is with many of the documents I recommend.

I found the most effective way to provide ready access to current documents securely is to password protect the documents on your computer, then put them in the cloud. Share them and your password only with family members. In case of an emergency, they could easily access the documents and use the password to open them in minutes. I save all changes to these documents on my computer and the cloud as they are made, so they are instantly up to date.

I also use Norton's Password Manager because it is convenient for opening accounts when on the computer. I use a relatively complex password to open

Password Manager which has to be entered to start each session. That password is included in the Passwords documents previously discussed.

Immediate access to financial records is not required, but if you have a financial spreadsheet document like mine, I recommend it be password protected and put in the cloud. Access to Morningstar is available on any computer by using your password. Access to your computer and your password is also required to use Quicken.

External drives are another option for providing access to documents. If you use them, explain where they are located and what is on them.

It is important to choose one or more of the methods described above. As the documents are prepared, make them available immediately. Make sure everyone who needs access to them knows how to do that.

Many of you might have had to handle the estate of a deceased family member. Think how much easier that would have been if the steps recommended in this section had been completed ahead of time. Your heirs will then be less stressed when dealing with your estate and be grateful for your preparation.

Acknowledgments

I never had any intention of writing a book. Writing a memoir for my family was the only writing I had done that was remotely related. It was a comment by my daughter, Kris Ann Carswell, that led to the creation of this book. If anyone gets to benefit from reading this book, they can thank my daughter.

I didn't take her suggestion seriously until I mentioned it to William (Bill) Huber, a high school friend and author of *Adolph Sutro: King of the Comstock Lode and Mayor of San Francisco*. He agreed with her suggestion and strongly encouraged me to write the book. Bill guided me through the process and continually encouraged me by telling me that I was writing a valuable book. He was very helpful throughout the process. He also reviewed the chapters as I wrote them, providing many useful ideas and editing suggestions. He was a great source of information about the multitude of things a first-time author needs to know to write a professional book.

My sister-in-law, Nancy Cover Reed, and brother, Frank Eden Reed, worked as a team while reviewing the book. Nancy, a teacher, suggested most of the edits. Frank offered his own and created the "track changes" document for my review. They also made uplifting comments about the importance and quality of the material, something I needed as a new author. Frank saved email messages that I had sent about key events as I progressed through changes in my capabilities and found solutions to them, which allowed me to construct a timeline of key events. Nancy made a significant, unexpected contribution when she surprised me with an attachment to an email titled "Don't Leave—An Ode to a Caregiver." It had a great impact on me and everyone else who read it. There is no doubt that the book is much better as a result of their contributions.

Fred Bowman, a fraternity brother and close friend since college, played vital roles as well. He didn't read the book as an editor. Instead, he made insightful, encouraging comments about the value of the subject matter and its likely effects on readers.

Dave Cowles, a fraternity brother, also reviewed the entire book and offered constructive suggestions that improved the book. His encouraging words were very helpful throughout this process.

Our son, Michael Alan Reed, reviewed those chapters that included very candid information about his mother's behavior and my potentially controversial approaches to deal with them. He said that since I was writing a book to help others, I had to be candid and agreed that this information should be included. He asked whether I was writing a storybook or a resource book. When I told him it was both, he suggested that I add a table at the front of the chapters on motorized scooters and motorized wheelchairs to enable the reader to see at a glance which device was better for each important consideration, e.g., safety.

More important than the quality of the writing is the content. The experiences that my wife and I had provided relevant content. So did the many references that I have included in the book, particularly those books by authors who experienced severe challenges of their own or who were caregivers for such people.

But I wanted first-hand information from people who went through the types of challenges that the readers were facing or were likely to face in the future. Here is where I got significant help from my fraternity brothers. Many of them or their wives had faced difficulties of their own. They saw the potential value of helping others by sharing their stories with me. They freely described their challenges and how they dealt with them. Multiple quotes from them are included in this book. I want to thank Fred Hellrich, Larry Haack, Bob Lindsay, Dick Hamme and Dave Cowles for helping me gain more insight on a variety of challenges they faced and the approaches they took to deal with them. Many other members of the fraternity encouraged me to write the book as well.

Fred Hellrich helped in multiple ways. When I faced a challenging, short-term move, he suggested an organization that would be helpful. Through that lead, I found someone that was crucial in accomplishing the move on time. He also suggested a way to self-publish if I had trouble finding a publisher. He reviewed those chapters where he had information that would be helpful and offered suggestions. His wife had experience rehabbing in a nursing home and later a continuing care retirement community (CCRC). He and his wife also had researched some potential senior living facilities, which allowed him to provide valuable content regarding senior care facilities that I included in Appendix I.

Bob Bailey, the Executive Director of LivGenerations Ahwatukee, and Pamela Brown, Director of Sales from Sunrise of Chandler, helped me understand the different ways in which senior living facilities determine assisted living care levels, which enabled me to share that information in the book.

Bob Bailey showed a keen interest in my book and told me he wanted to help. Among the many things he did was to introduce me to Dr. Marwan Sabbagh who wrote the Foreword to this book.

The encouragement I got from my extended family, friends and neighbors, along with the very favorable comments they made about the excerpts I shared with them, encouraged me to continue this work.

I want to thank my wife, Joan Derby Reed, for understanding why she didn't get as much attention as she should have when I spent so many hours day and night working on the book.

All of the previous acknowledgments were related to the book's creation. But my goal was to help as many people as possible. As a first-time author, I needed someone recognized as an expert to validate the content. I am honored to have had the eminent Dr. Marwan Sabbagh take time out of his busy schedule to write the Foreword of this book.

Chapter Notes

Chapter 1

1. NIH National Institute of Neurological Disorders and Stroke. 2019. "Peripheral Neuropathy Fact Sheet." August 13. Accessed November 25, 2019. https://www.ninds.nih.gov/Disorders/Patient-Caregiver-Education/Fact-Sheets/Peripheral-Neuropathy-Fact-Sheet.

2. Muscular Dystrophy Association. 2019. "Inclusion-Body Myositis (IBM)." Accessed November 25, 2019. https://www.mda.org/disease/inclusion-body-myositis.

3. Cleveland Clinic. 2019. "Inclusion Body Myositis." Accessed November 25, 2019. https://my.clevelandclinic.org/health/diseases/15700-inclusion-body-myositis.

4. Muscular Dystrophy Association, op. cit.

Chapter 2

1. Kübler-Ross, Elisabeth. 1969. *On Death and Dying*. New York: Scribner.

2. Jackson, Kate. 2014. "Grieving Chronic Illness and Injury—Infinite Losses." *Social Work Today*, July/August: 18.

3. Wolfelt, Jaimie A., Alan D. Wolfelt. 2019. *Healing Your Chronic Illness Grief: 100 Practical Ideas for Living Your Best Life*. Fort Collins: Companion Press.

4. Family Caregiver Alliance; reviewed by Rabbi Jon Sommer. 1996, 2013. "Grief and Loss." Family Caregiver Alliance, National Center on Caregiving. Accessed August 24, 2019. https://www.caregiver.org/grief-and-loss.

Chapter 4

1. Carpenter, Leanna. 2019. "How Muscles Get Big: The Science Behind Muscle Soreness and Building Muscle Mass." Weight Watchers International, Inc. Accessed August 24, 2019. https://www.weightwatchers.ca/util/art/index_art.aspx?tabnum=1&art_id=134551&sc=3039.

Chapter 9

1. United Spinal Association. 2019. "Types of Wheelchairs—A Visual Tour." Accessed September 2, 2019. http://www.unitedspinal.org/disability-products-services/types-of-wheelchairs/.

2. Mobility Management. 2010. "How to Choose the Best Power Chair Drive Configuration." Mobility Management. Accessed September 2, 2019. https://mobilitymgmt.com/articles/2010/07/01/power-chair-drive.aspx.

3. Wechsler, Kathy. 2011. "Front, Middle or Rear? Finding the Power Chair Drive System That's Right for You." Muscular Dystrophy Association. Accessed September 2, 2019. https://www.mda.org/quest/article/front-middle-or-rear-finding-power-chair-drive-system-thats-right-you.

4. EZ Lock Incorporated. 2019. "Welcome to EZ Lock!" Accessed September 4, 2019. http://www.ezlock.net/.

5. Mobility Basics, ca. 2002–2019. "Power Wheelchair Drive Controls." Accessed September 2, 2019. https://mobilitybasics.ca/wheelchairs/drivecontrols.

6. Invacare. 2019. "The Application of Power Tilt, Recline, and Power Elevating Legs and How They Assist with Pressure, Positioning, and Function." Invacare. Accessed September 2, 2019. https://www.passionatepeople.invacare.eu.com/power-tilt-recline-and-power-elevating-legs-pressure-positioning/.

7. Hoveround. 2013. "Power Wheelchair Cushion Types." Hoveround. June 3. Accessed September 2, 2019. https://www.hoveround.com/articles/wheelchair-cushion-types.

Chapter 10

1. Tablebases.com. 2011. "Accessible Dining, Banquet and Bar Tables and Bases." Tablebases.com. November 18. Accessed September 2, 2019. https://tablebases.com/blog/2011/11/accessible-dining-banquet-and-bar-tables-and-bases/.

2. Louie, Emma. 2017. "Tips for Dining Out in a Wheelchair." Karman. August 14. Accessed September 2, 2019. https://www.karmanhealthcare.com/tips-dining/.

3. Edward. 2018. "How Much Does It Cost to Repair a Wheelchair Motor?" Karman. December 5. Accessed September 2, 2019. https://www.

karmanhealthcare.com/how-much-does-it-cost-to-repair-a-wheelchair-motor/.

Chapter 11

1. Havens, Brian. 2015. "Does Medicare Cover Stair Lifts? What You Need to Know About Stair Lift Funding" 101Mobility. September 2. Accessed September 3, 2019. https://101mobility.com/blog/how-to-find-stair-lift-funding/.

Chapter 12

1. Smart911. 2019. "Smart911 Saves Time and Saves Lives." Accessed September 19, 2019. https://safety.smart911.com/how-it-works.

2. Roberts, Catherine. 2019. "How to Choose a Medical Alert System." Consumer Reports. February 7. Accessed August 28, 2019. https://www.consumerreports.org/medical-alert-systems/how-to-choose-a-medical-alert-system/.

3. Knox Company. 2019. "Home Emergency Access." Accessed September 19, 2019. https://www.knoxbox.com/Products/Residential-KnoxBoxes.

4. Consumer Reports. 2019. "Generator Buying Guide." August 28. Accessed September 23, 2019. https://www.consumerreports.org/cro/generators/buying-guide/index.htm.

Chapter 14

1. Nuprodx Mobility. 2019. "State of the Art in Mobility." Accessed September 2019. https://www.nuprodx.com/.

Chapter 16

1. Celiac Disease Foundation. 2019. "What Is Celiac Disease?" Accessed September 8, 2019. https://celiac.org/about-celiac-disease/what-is-celiac-disease/.

2. Permutter, David, M.D. 2019. "Gluten Containing Products." Accessed September 8, 2019. https://www.drperlmutter.com/eat/foods-that-contain-gluten/.

Chapter 19

1. National Aging and Disability Transportation Center. 2019. "ADA and Paratransit: What Is ADA Complementary Paratransit?" Accessed October 7, 2019. https://www.nadtc.org/about/transportation-aging-disability/ada-and-paratransit/.

Chapter 20

1. Ability Center. 2018. "Driving Aids." Accessed December 3, 2019. https://www.abilitycenter.com/mobility-products/driving-aids/.

2. Adapt Solutions. 2018. "What Is Your Solution?" Adapt Solutions. Accessed December 8, 2019. https://adaptsolutions.com/products/.

3. Sure Grip Hand Controls. 2019. "Switch." Sure Grip. Accessed December 8, 2019. https://www.suregrip-handcontrols.com/switch.

Chapter 21

1. McGivney, Monique. 2015. "Types of Driving Aids and Hand Controls." Ability Center. September 1. Accessed December 3, 2019. https://www.abilitycenter.com/types-of-driving-aids-and-hand-controls/.

Chapter 26

1. TenNapel Tyrone, Jamie, and Dr. Marwan Noel Sabbagh. 2019. *Fighting for My Life: How to Thrive in the Shadow of Alzheimer's*. New York: HarperCollins.

2. *Ibid.*

3. *Ibid.*

4. Mace, Nancy L., and Peter V. Rabins, M.D., MPH. 2017. *The 36-Hour Day: A Family Guide to Caring for People Who Have Alzheimer Disease, Other Dementias, and Memory Loss*. Baltimore: Johns Hopkins University Press.

5. Alzheimer's Association. 2020. "Facts and Figures." Alzheimer's Association. Accessed February 13, 2020. https://www.alz.org/alzheimers-dementia/facts-figures.

6. Alzheimer's Association. 2019. "2019 Alzheimer's Disease Facts and Figures." Alzheimer's Association. Accessed February 15, 2020. https://www.alz.org/media/Documents/alzheimers-facts-and-figures-2019-r.pdf.

7. Robinson, Lawrence, Melissa S. Wayne, M.A., and Jeanne Segal, Ph.D. 2019. "Alzheimer's and Dementia Care: Help for Family Caregivers" HelpGuide, Your Trusted Guide to Mental Health and Wellness. August. Accessed February 5, 2020. https://www.helpguide.org/articles/alzheimers-dementia-aging/tips-for-alzheimers-caregivers.htm.

8. Mayo Clinic. 2019. "Alzheimer's Stages: How the Disease Progresses." Mayo Clinic. May 7. Accessed February 5, 2020. https://www.mayoclinic.org/diseases-conditions/alzheimers-disease/in-depth/alzheimers-stages/art-20048448.

Chapter 27

1. Robinson, op. cit.

2. Mayo Clinic, op. cit.

3. National Institute on Aging. 2017. "Alzheimer's Caregiving: Changes in Communication Skills." National Institute on Aging. May 17. Accessed February 5, 2020. https://www.nia.nih.gov/health/alzheimers-caregiving-changes-communication-skills.

4. Mayo Clinic, op. cit.
5. National Institute on Aging, op. cit.
6. Mayo Clinic, op. cit.
7. Reed, Tara. 2015. *What to do Between the Tears: A Practical Guide to Dealing with a Dementia or Alzheimer's Diagnosis in the Family.* Tigard, OR: Pivot to Happy Press.
8. *Ibid.*
9. Mayo Clinic, op. cit.
10. Robinson, op. cit.

Chapter 28

1. National Institute on Aging, op. cit.
2. Neighmond, Patti. 2019. "Her Mom Was Lost in Dementia's Fog. Singing Christmas Carols Brought Her Back." NPR. December 24. Accessed February 6, 2020. https://www.npr.org/sections/health-shots/2019/12/24/790806366/her-mom-was-lost-in-dementias-fog-singing-christmas-carols-brought-her-back.
3. Oh, Jeewon, William J. Chopik, and Eric S. Kim. 2019. "The Association Between Actor/Partner Optimism and Cognitive Functioning Among Older Couples." *Journal of Personality.* November 29: 1–11.
4. *Ibid.*
5. Sauer, Alissa. 2014. "Laughter for Alzheimer's Prevention." August 14. Accessed February 14, 2020. https://www.alzheimers.net/8-13-14-laughter-and-alzheimers/.
6. *Ibid.*
7. *Ibid.*
8. Robinson, op. cit.
9. Christiansen, Sherry. n.d. "Can Specially Trained Dogs Help People with Alzheimer's Dementia?" Accessed February 14, 2020. https://www.alzu.org/blog/2017/05/30/how-service-dogs-can-help-people-with-alzheimers-dementia/.
10. *Ibid.*
11. National Institute on Aging, op. cit.

Chapter 29

1. National Institute on Aging, op. cit.
2. Drugs.com. 2019. "Quetiapine Tablets." Drugs.com. September 11. Accessed February 8, 2020. https://www.drugs.com/cdi/quetiapine-tablets.html.

Appendix I

1. National Institue on Aging. 2017. "Residential Facilities, Assisted Living, and Nursing Homes." National Institute on Aging. May 1. Accessed May 24, 2020. https://www.nia.nih.gov/health/residential-facilities-assisted-living-and-nursing-homes.
2. Ecker, Elizabeth. 2018. "Largest Senior Living Provider List Grows in 2018." Senior Housing News. October 17. Accessed June 5, 2020. https://seniorhousingnews.com/2018/10/17/largest-senior-living-provider-list-grows-2018/.
3. Argentum. 2020. "Expanding Senior Living." Accessed June 5, 2020. https://www.argentum.org/.

Appendix II

1. National Association of Insurance Commissioners. 2019. "A Shopper's Guide to Long-Term Care Insurance." National Association of Insurance Commissioners. Accessed April 5, 2020. https://www.naic.org/documents/prod_serv_consumer_ltc_lp.pdf.
2. New York Life Insurance Company. 2020. "Long-Term Care: Plan for the Future." Accessed May 23, 2020. https://www.nylaarp.com/Landing-Pages/LongTermCare?tntph=PPCLTC9053&cid=3R1W3O&mkwid=sOy042fDLdc_pcrid_252904721640_pmt_e_pkw_long%20term%20care%20insurance&gclid=-EAIaIQobChMIyPv-q-_K6QIVrx6tBh2hZQGUEAAYASAAEgIjP_D_BwE.
3. Marquand, Barbara. 2019. "Long-Term Care Insurance Explained." NerdWallet. May 29. Accessed March 5, 2020. https://www.nerdwallet.com/blog/insurance/long-term-care-insurance/.
4. Favreault, Melissa, and Judith Dey. 2016. "Long-Term Services and Supports for Older Americans: Risks and Financing Research Brief." U.S. Department of Health and Human Services. Accessed May 23, 2020. https://aspe.hhs.gov/basic-report/long-term-services-and-supports-older-americans-risks-and-financing-research-brief.
5. Stark, Ellen. 2018. "5 Things You SHOULD Know About Long-Term Care Insurance." Family Caregiving: Financial and Legal. March 1. Accessed May 23, 2020. https://www.aarp.org/caregiving/financial-legal/info-2018/long-term-care-insurance-fd.html.
6. *Ibid.*
7. Genworth Financial, Inc. 2020. "Cost of Care Survey 2019." Accessed March 5, 2020. https://www.genworth.com/aging-and-you/finances/cost-of-care.html.

Appendix III

1. Korving, Arie J. 2002. *Before I Go: Preparing Your Affairs for Your Heirs.* Suffolk: Korving & Company LLC.
2. Miller, B.J., and Shoshana Berger. 2019. *A Beginner's Guide to the End: Practical Advice for Living Life and Facing Death.* New York: Simon & Shuster.
3. *Ibid.*

Bibliography

Ability Center. 2018. "Driving Aids." Accessed December 3, 2019. https://www.abilitycenter.com/mobility-products/driving-aids/.

Adapt Solutions. 2018. "What Is Your Solution?" Adapt Solutions. Accessed December 8, 2019. https://adaptsolutions.com/products/.

Alzheimer's Association. 2019. "2019 Alzheimer's Disease Facts and Figures." Alzheimer's Association. Accessed February 15, 2020. https://www.alz.org/media/Documents/alzheimers-facts-and-figures-2019-r.pdf.

Alzheimer's Association. 2020. "Facts and Figures." Alzheimer's Association. Accessed February 13, 2020. https://www.alz.org/alzheimers-dementia/facts-figures.

Carpenter, Leanna. 2019. "How Muscles Get Big: The Science Behind Muscle Soreness and Building Muscle Mass." Weight Watchers International, Inc. Accessed August 24, 2019. https://www.weightwatchers.ca/util/art/index_art.aspx?tabnum=1&art_id=134551&sc=3039.

Celiac Disease Foundation. 2019. "What Is Celiac Disease?" Accessed September 8, 2019. https://celiac.org/about-celiac-disease/what-is-celiac-disease/#.

Christiansen, Sherry. n.d. "Can Specially Trained Dogs Help People with Alzheimer's Dementia?" Alzheimer's Universe. Accessed February 14, 2020. https://www.alzu.org/blog/2017/05/30/how-service-dogs-can-help-people-with-alzheimers-dementia/.

Cleveland Clinic. 2019. "Inclusion Body Myositis." Accessed November 25, 2019. https://my.clevelandclinic.org/health/diseases/15700-inclusion-body-myositis.

Consumer Reports. 2019. "Generator Buying Guide." August 28. Accessed September 23, 2019. https://www.consumerreports.org/cro/generators/buying-guide/index.htm.

Demmitt, Audrey, R.N. 2020. "Ten Tips for Caregivers of Individuals with Vision Loss." VisionAware. Accessed February 14, 2020. https://visionaware.org/emotional-support/for-family-and-friends/guidance-for-caregivers-of-individuals-who-are-blind-or-visually-impaired/ten-tips-for-caregivers-of-individuals-with-vision-loss/.

Drugs.com. 2019. "Quetiapine Tablets." Drugs.com. September 11. Accessed February 8, 2020. https://www.drugs.com/cdi/quetiapine-tablets.html.

Ecker, Elizabeth. 2018. "Largest Senior Living Provider List Grows in 2018." Senior Housing News. October 17. Accessed June 5, 2020. https://seniorhousingnews.com/2018/10/17/largest-senior-living-provider-list-grows-2018/.

Edward. 2018. "How Much Does It Cost to Repair a Wheelchair Motor?" Karman. December 5. Accessed September 2, 2019. https://www.karmanhealthcare.com/how-much-does-it-cost-to-repair-a-wheelchair-motor/.

EZ Lock Incorporated. 2019. "Welcome to EZ Lock!" Accessed September 4, 2019. http://www.ezlock.net/.

Family Caregiver Alliance; reviewed by Rabbi Jon Sommer. 1996, 2013. "Grief and Loss." Family Caregiver Alliance, National Center on Caregiving. Accessed August 24, 2019. https://www.caregiver.org/grief-and-loss.

Favreault, Melissa, and Judith Dey. 2016. "Long-Term Services and Supports for Older Americans: Risks and Financing Research Brief." U.S. Department of Health and Human Services. Accessed May 23, 2020. https://aspe.hhs.gov/basic-report/long-term-services-and-supports-older-americans-risks-and-financing-research-brief.

Genworth Financial, Inc. 2020. "Cost of Care Survey 2019." Accessed March 5, 2020. https://www.genworth.com/aging-and-you/finances/cost-of-care.html.

Havens, Brian. 2015. "Does Medicare Cover Stair Lifts? What You Need to Know About Stair Lift Funding" 101Mobility. September 2. Accessed September 3, 2019. https://101mobility.com/blog/how-to-find-stair-lift-funding/.

Hoveround. 2013. "Power Wheelchair Cushion Types." Hoveround. June 3. Accessed September 2, 2019. https://www.hoveround.com/articles/wheelchair-cushion-types.

Invacare. 2019. "The Application of Power Tilt, Recline and Power Elevating Legs and How They Assist with Pressure, Positioning and

Function." Invacare. Accessed September 2, 2019. https://www.passionatepeople.invacare.eu.com/power-tilt-recline-and-power-elevating-legs-pressure-positioning/.

Jackson, Kate. 2014. "Grieving Chronic Illness and Injury—Infinite Losses." *Social Work Today,* July/August: 18.

Knox Company. 2019. "Home Emergency Access." Accessed September 19, 2019. https://www.knoxbox.com/Products/Residential-KnoxBoxes.

Korving, Arie J. 2002. *Before I Go: Preparing Your Affairs for Your Heirs.* Suffolk: Korving & Company LLC.

Kübler-Ross, Elisabeth. 1969. *On Death and Dying.* New York: Scribner.

Louie, Emma. 2017. "Tips for Dining Out in a Wheelchair." Karman. August 14. Accessed September 2, 2019. https://www.karmanhealthcare.com/tips-dining/.

Marquand, Barbara. 2019. "Long-Term Care Insurance Explained." NerdWallet. May 29. Accessed March 5, 2020. https://www.nerdwallet.com/blog/insurance/long-term-care-insurance/.

Mayo Clinic. 2019. "Alzheimer's and Dementia Care: Tips for Daily Tasks." Mayo Clinic. May 7. Accessed February 5, 2020.

Mayo Clinic Staff. 2019. "Alzheimer's Stages: How the Disease Progresses." April 19. Accessed April 29, 2020. https://www.mayoclinic.org/diseases-conditions/alzheimers-disease/in-depth/alzheimers-stages/art-20048448.

McGivney, Monique. 2015. "Types of Driving Aids and Hand Controls." Ability Center. September 1. Accessed December 3, 2019. https://www.abilitycenter.com/types-of-driving-aids-and-hand-controls/.

Miller, B.J., and Shoshana Berger. 2019. *A Beginner's Guide to the End: Practical Advice for Living Life and Facing Death.* New York: Simon & Schuster.

Mobility Basics, ca. 2002–2019. "Power Wheelchair Drive Controls." Accessed September 2, 2019. https://mobilitybasics.ca/wheelchairs/drivecontrols.

Mobility Management. 2010. "How to Choose the Best Power Chair Drive Configuration." Mobility Management. July 1. Accessed September 2, 2019. https://mobilitymgmt.com/articles/2010/07/01/power-chair-drive.aspx.

Muscular Dystrophy Association. 2019. "Inclusion-Body Myositis (IBM)." Accessed November 25, 2019. https://www.mda.org/disease/inclusion-body-myositis.

National Aging and Disability Transportation Center. 2019. "ADA and Paratransit: What Is ADA Complementary Paratransit?" Accessed October 7, 2019. https://www.nadtc.org/about/transportation-aging-disability/ada-and-paratransit/.

National Association of Insurance Commissioners. 2019. "A Shopper's Guide to Long-Term Care Insurance." National Association of Insurance Commissioners. Accessed April 5, 2020. https://www.naic.org/documents/prod_serv_consumer_ltc_lp.pdf.

National Institute on Aging. 2017. "Alzheimer's Caregiving: Changes in Communication Skills." National Institute on Aging. May 17. Accessed February 5, 2020. https://www.nia.nih.gov/health/alzheimers-caregiving-changes-communication-skills.

_____. 2017. "Residential Facilities, Assisted Living, and Nursing Homes." National Institute on Aging. May 1. Accessed May 24, 2020. https://www.nia.nih.gov/health/residential-facilities-assisted-living-and-nursing-homes.

Neighmond, Patti. 2019. "Her Mom Was Lost in Dementia's Fog. Singing Christmas Carols Brought Her Back." NPR. December 24. Accessed February 6, 2020. https://www.npr.org/sections/health-shots/2019/12/24/790806366/her-mom-was-lost-in-dementias-fog-singing-christmas-carols-brought-her-back.

New York Life Insurance Company. 2020. "Long-Term Care: Plan for the Future." Accessed May 23, 2020. https://www.nylaarp.com/Landing-Pages/LongTermCare?tntph=PPCLTC9053&cid=3R1W3O&mkwid=sOy042fDL-dc_pcrid_252904721640_pmt_e_pkw_long%20term%20care%20insurance&gclid=-EAIaIQobChMIyPv-q-_K6QIVrx6tBh2hZQGUEAAYASAAEgIjP_D_BwE.

NIH National Institute of Neurological Disorders and Stroke. 2019. "Peripheral Neuropathy Fact Sheet." August 13. Accessed November 25, 2019. https://www.ninds.nih.gov/Disorders/Patient-Caregiver-Education/Fact-Sheets/Peripheral-Neuropathy-Fact-Sheet.

Nuprodx Mobility. 2019. "State of the Art in Mobility." Accessed September 2019. https://www.nuprodx.com/.

Oh, Jeewon, William J. Chopik, and Eric S. Kim. 2019. "The Association Between Actor/Partner Optimism and Cognitive Functioning Among Older Couples." *Journal of Personality.* November 29: 1–11.

Permutter, David, M.D. 2019. "Gluten Containing Products." Accessed September 8, 2019. https://www.drperlmutter.com/eat/foods-that-contain-gluten/.

Reed, Tara. 2015. *What to do Between the Tears: A Practical Guide to Dealing with a Dementia or Alzheimer's Diagnosis in the Family.* Tigard, OR: Pivot to Happy Press.

Roberts, Catherine. 2019. "How to Choose a Medical Alert System." Consumer Reports. February 7. Accessed August 28, 2019. https://www.consumerreports.org/medical-alert-systems/how-to-choose-a-medical-alert-system/.

Robinson, Lawrence, Melissa S. Wayne, M.A., and Jeanne Segal, Ph.D. 2019. "Tips for Alzheimer's and Dementia Caregivers." HelpGuide, Your Trusted Guide to Mental Health and Wellness. August. Accessed February 5, 2020. https://www.helpguide.org/

articles/alzheimers-dementia-aging/tips-for-alzheimers-caregivers.htm.

Sauer, Alissa. 2014. "Laughter for Alzheimer's Prevention." Alzheimers.net. August 14. Accessed February 14, 2020. https://www.alzheimers.net/8-13-14-laughter-and-alzheimers/.

Smart911. 2019. "Smart911 Saves Time and Saves Lives." Accessed September 19, 2019. https://safety.smart911.com/how-it-works.

Stark, Ellen. 2018. "5 Things You SHOULD Know About Long-Term Care Insurance." Family Caregiving: Financial and Legal. March 1. Accessed May 23, 2020. https://www.aarp.org/caregiving/financial-legal/info-2018/long-term-care-insurance-fd.html.

Sure Grip Hand Controls. 2019. "Switch." Sure Grip. Accessed December 8, 2019. https://www.suregrip-handcontrols.com/switch.

Tablebases.com. 2011. "Accessible Dining, Banquet and Bar Tables and Bases." Tablebases.com. November 18. Accessed September 2, 2019. https://tablebases.com/blog/2011/11/accessible-dining-banquet-and-bar-tables-and-bases/.

TenNapel Tyrone, Jamie, and Dr. Marwan Noel Sabbagh. 2019. *Fighting for My Life: How to Thrive in the Shadow of Alzheimer's.* New York: HarperCollins.

United Spinal Association. 2019. "Types of Wheelchairs—A Visual Tour." Accessed September 2, 2019. http://www.unitedspinal.org/disability-products-services/types-of-wheelchairs/.

WebMD Medical Reference Reviewed by Neil Lava, MD. 2018. "Coping Tips for Caregivers of Those with Parkinson's Disease." WebMD. November 11. Accessed February 14, 2020. https://www.webmd.com/parkinsons-disease/guide/parkinsons-caregivers#1.

Wechsler, Kathy. 2011. "Front, Middle or Rear? Finding the Power Chair Drive System That's Right for You." Muscular Dystrophy Association. September 30. Accessed September 2, 2019. https://www.mda.org/quest/article/front-middle-or-rear-finding-power-chair-drive-system-thats-right-you.

Wolfelt, Jaimie A., and Alan D. Wolfelt. 2019. *Healing Your Chronic Illness Grief: 100 Practical Ideas for Living Your Best Life.* Fort Collins: Companion Press.

Index